# Cancer and Radiotherapy

*By the same author*
with H. Miller, M.A., Ph.D., F.Inst.P.

**A Short Textbook of Radiotherapy**
**for Technicians and Students**

# Cancer and Radiotherapy

## A Short Guide for Nurses and Medical Students

**J. WALTER** M.A., B.M. (Oxon), F.R.C.P., F.R.C.R.,
D.M.R.E. (Camb.)

Consultant Radiotherapist, Weston Park Hospital, Sheffield;
Hon. Clinical Lecturer in Radiotherapy, University of Sheffield.

Second edition

CHURCHILL LIVINGSTONE
EDINBURGH LONDON. AND NEW YORK 1977

CHURCHILL LIVINGSTONE
Medical Division of Longman Group Limited

Distributed in the United States of America by Longman Inc.,
19 West 44th Street, New York, N.Y. 10036 and by associated
companies, branches and representatives throughout the world.

© Longman Group Limited, 1977

First edition 1971
  Reprinted 1973
Second edition 1977

ISBN 0 443 01533 3

Library of Congress Cataloging in Publication Data
Walter, Joseph, physician.
  Cancer and radiotherapy.

  Bibliography: p. 265
  Includes index.
  1. Cancer—Radiotherapy.  2. Cancer.  I. Title.
[DNLM:  1. Neoplasms—Radiotherapy.  QZ269 W232c]
RC271.R3W3  1977    616.9′94′0642    76-28431

Printed in Singapore

To
**Oliver and Leonor**

*'Tis the good reader that makes the good book.'*

Emerson

*'A book is a machine for thinking with.'*

I. A. Richards

# Preface to Second edition

The concept of 'Oncology' is now widely accepted, and we hear of 'oncological nursing' etc. For this edition alterations and additions have been made in every chapter. There are new sections on the acute radiation syndrome, cancer of the prostate and retinoblastoma, and considerable amendments on cancer in children. Advances in lymphoreticular disorders (Hodgkin's disease, leukaemia etc.) have led me to expand on these and separate them into a new additional chapter.

The most active sector of the oncological front is now cytotoxic chemotherapy. I have brought this fairly up-to-date, but it is neither necessary nor desirable (nor possible) to include every single new drug. There is far too much ill-advised cytotoxic therapy now practised, mainly for the sake of 'doing something' and just because the drugs are available. I have therefore pitched my enthusiasm in a lower key than that of some ardent advocates.

I am grateful for the criticisms and comments on the first edition. I have firmly resisted suggestions to introduce more technicalities (e.g. on cell kinetics) suitable for (some) medical students but not for (most) nurses. I am again indebted to several colleagues for specialised help, including Dr F. E. Neal, who has revised the section on iodine and the thyroid, Dr I. G. Emmanuel, Dr J. S. L. Lilleyman and Mr K. Bomford.

Sheffield, 1977

J. W.

# Preface to the First edition

This little book has been written to fill a gap. It is an expansion of lectures given over the years to junior and senior nurses at general and radiotherapy hospitals, as well as on the 'district'.

The title might well have been *Oncology* (study and management of tumours), a useful word that is beginning to come into use but is still unfamiliar. I have tried to deal with most aspects, including public health (prevention, education etc.), but not surgical management which is very adequately dealt with elsewhere and would be out of place here. Oncology is visibly fragmenting with the inevitable onrush of super-specialisation. Surgeons have long been a breed apart. The radiotherapist began almost as a technical assistant but progressed, almost against his own will, to approximate more and more to the 'compleat oncologist'. Now we have – or are in process of acquiring – full-time practitioners of nuclear medicine (isotopes), cytotoxic chemotherapy and (soon) immunotherapy. The day may not be far off when no one person would think of attempting to cover the whole field above an elementary level.

The main emphasis is on radiotherapy. I hope I have given enough – but not too much – physics (a subject anathema to many, not excepting doctors) to make the scientific and practical basis intelligible. Medical oncology has been included – i.e. hormones and cytotoxic drugs. Most radiotherapists (at least in Britain) find themselves obliged to gather some expertise in this field also, and a radiotherapy ward may have an appreciable proportion of patients undergoing such therapy.

The book is designed primarily for nurses. I hope that much of it will interest any nurse at any stage of her career, but it should be of most use to the experienced nurse fresh to a radiotherapy ward or department. I have included medical students in the title. Although part of the contents will be elementary for them, they may find it useful to have a collected account of a subject which is usually fragmented, including some aspects they might not readily find elsewhere and often omitted from their curriculum. If it leads a few to consider taking up this outlandish speciality, it would be gratifying.

I hope it may also be of interest to ancillary workers such as radiographers, physicists, biochemists, laboratory and social workers. Comments, criticisms and suggestions will be welcomed.

I am grateful to various authors and publishers for permission to use illustrations etc.; these are individually acknowledged. I would also like

to thank my publishers for their unfailing help, and their editor Mr R. A.
Lomax for his expert supervision and helpful suggestions.

**J. W.**

Weston Park Hospital
Whitham Road
Sheffield S10 2SJ.

# Contents

reactions, Mucous membranes, Blood-forming tissues, Reproductive organs, Eye, Kidney, Brain, Bone, Lung, Radiation sickness.

# 1. The Cancer Problem

*'Tis a mad world, my masters.*

John Taylor (1580-1653)

No nurse or doctor will need persuading of the importance and seriousness of cancer. It is the second most important cause of death in western countries — one in five deaths is due to cancer.

To put it another way, *a quarter of all infants born in the U.K. will develop cancer* at some stage of their lives. Eighty per cent of these will die of it, 20 per cent will be cured.

Considerable fear and prejudice, much of it born of ignorance, surrounds the public image of cancer. The lay mind tends to associate cancer with pain, incurability and misery and this makes its management even more difficult for nurses and doctors. There are, of course, very

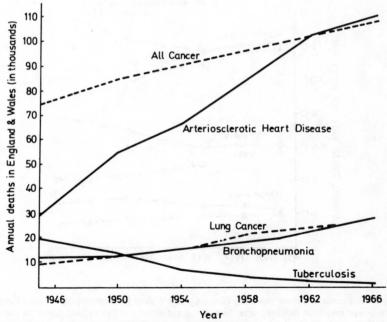

Fig. 1.1 Trends in mortality showing causes of death.

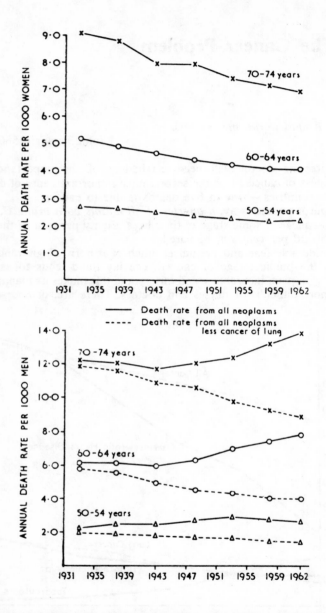

Fig. 1. 2. Trends in cancer mortality (England and Wales) for women (*upper graph*) and men (*lower graph*) at different ages. Note the great difference due to lung cancer in men. (*Courtesy Prof. R. Doll*)

good reasons for cancer's evil reputation, but the picture is not so black as it is often painted. There has been much progress in all aspects of the problem, so that we are now in a better position to cope with it than ever before.

## Cancer incidence

In spite of its importance as a cause of death, cancer is not a common disease. A general practitioner, with 3500 patients on his list, will sign on average 40 death certificates a year, of which eight will have cancer as the primary cause. In a large general hospital less than 5 per cent of admissions will be for cancer. Compare this with a radiotherapy ward where nearly every patient will have malignant disease. There is a relatively high incidence in geriatric and terminal care units too.

Overall about three new cases are seen annually per thousand of population, so that a city of one million will have some 3000 new cases per year. It is worth noting that rather *more than half of these will be treated by some form of radiotherapy* at some stage.

In particular age groups, especially 50-60 and 60-70, cancer mortality is not increasing. A notable exception is lung cancer. In some instances it has fallen − e.g. mouth, stomach, uterus. It is only the grand total that has increased and this is because the population is becoming bigger and living longer. Naturally this imposes a growing strain on nursing and medical services.

The diagram below contrasts the current incidence of cancer at various common sites in the body. Although figures refer to this country, the picture is much the same in North America.

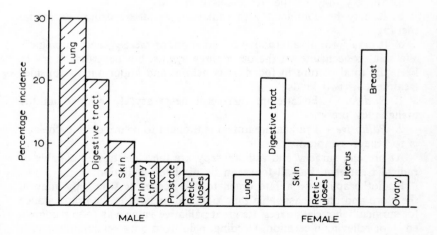

Fig. 1.3 Commonest cancers (England and Wales).

All of these except the reticuloses are *carcinomas*. Carcinomas account for 70-75 per cent of all cancers.

We shall deal with most of these groups in later chapters, but will have little to say about cancers of the gastro-intestinal tract since here radiation has only a minor part to play. In this group, till recently, the commonest site was the stomach, but gastric cancer is now declining and colon cancer is now rather commoner. In fact, cancer of the large bowel is now the second commonest lethal cancer in Britain, only exceeded by lung cancer. Next comes cancer of the rectum, followed by the pancreas. In contrast, oesophageal carcinoma is rare.

The picture presented in Fig. 1.3 is not a static one. The frequency of cancer and its relative incidence at different sites show considerable variations between different countries, different social classes, different cultural and educational groups, different environments (urban, rural, industrial etc.) and therefore will change from decade to decade even in the same country. Compared with the early years of this century, we find more leukaemia and cancer of the lung and bladder in England today, but less of the stomach, bowel and mouth.

## The management of cancer

Management means care. It also means prevention, early detection and education. When a case has been diagnosed, we have four specific modes of treatment at our disposal:

1. *Surgery*        3. *Hormones*
2. *Radiotherapy*   4. *Cytotoxic drugs*

This book will not concern itself with surgical treatment, except to indicate its role in certain types of cancer.

a. Surgery may be the treatment of choice.

b. It may be combined with radiation, cytotoxic drugs, hormonal therapy.

c. It may form an alternative to radiation, or merely serve to palliate. We shall concentrate on the other three agents, but nevertheless try to keep the total picture in focus. It is helpful and important to consider treatment as two kinds:

1. *Radical* – the attempt, heroic if necessary, to remove all the malignancy present.

2. *Palliative* – if radical treatment is thought to be impossible, the aim is to relieve symptoms.

At present, surgery and radiotherapy are the chief agents capable of radical treatment, but all four can be used for palliation.

Radiotherapy was a latecomer to the scene. It was only natural therefore and only reasonable that it should be used in the first instance for surgically hopeless cases. Its great palliative value was soon recognised – for relieving ulceration, bleeding, pain from bone secondaries etc. It was so successful, in fact, that its potential in radical treatment was overshadowed, and it became psychologically associated with inoperable, incurable cancer. Something of this reputation still lingers, but it should now be clearly recognised that *radiotherapy stands on its own feet as a curative agent comparable to surgery, and capable of giving results just as good (and often better) in properly selected cases.*

However there is sometimes a psychological advantage in the choice of surgery, even when radiation offers a sound alternative, e.g. early cancer of the cervix. This is because radiation is closely associated in the minds of many patients with malignancy. Surgery on the other hand covers a much wider field and may be preferred when it is particularly important to conceal the truth from an apprehensive patient.

The relative value and uses of the various agents will be discussed later. In many sites, surgery is definitely better. In others radiotherapy has been found to yield superior results, and a summary account is given on pp. 83-4. In some cases it is advisable to use a combination of agents:

1. *pre-operative radiation*     as described under breast cancer (p. 118)
2. *post-operative radiation*     and Wilms's tumour (p. 238)

In others, agents are best used in sequence:

  a. *the primary growth*
  b. *the secondary lymph-nodes.*

For example, in seminoma of testis, the primary is first removed by orchidectomy and the secondary nodes are then irradiated. In cancer of the tongue, the primary is first treated by radiation, and secondary nodes in the neck then removed by block dissection.

Hormones are usually reserved until the resources of surgery and radiotherapy have been exhausted. Till recently the same applied to cytotoxics, but these have now acquired a predominant role in some types of cancer (malignant lymphoma, childhood tumours, leukaemia etc.) where they become the sole treatment or an essential part of it.

### Prognosis in cancer: The concept of cure

We might have used the expression 'curative' instead of 'radical' treatment. 'Cure' seems simple enough. We know what we mean by cure of a simple fracture or of the common cold even though complications like sinusitis or pneumonia may follow. We mean restoration to health — more or less complete, and free from further trouble. But what do we mean by 'cure' of, say, diabetes or pernicious anaemia? We can usually hold them at bay for long periods of time, maybe till the patient dies a natural death from some other cause at a ripe old age. In other words we can usually control them well enough for the patient to lead a normal — or nearly normal — life. This often holds good for cancer, and *'control' is a better word than 'cure'.*

In many early cancer cases we can be fairly confident that we have eliminated all traces of malignancy, but we can never be sure. Local recurrence or distant metastasis (Greek for 'shift in position') is always a possibility. A notorious example is breast cancer, where late recurrence or metastasis can occur after many years, even after many decades. Another is melanoma of the choroid; many years after the removal of the eye, the patient may present with an enlarged liver full of secondaries. Such cases are exceptional, but by no means rare.

*Indices of success.* In measuring the success of treatment for cancer, a conventional 'yardstick' is the proportion of patients who survive for a certain number of years – usually five. *Five-year survival* figures give us valuable information about the results of different forms of treatment. But five-year survival is sometimes interpreted as 'cure' and this can be seriously misleading. In many cases, if a patient survives and is well after five years, his chances of remaining permanently free of malignancy are excellent, e.g. cancer of the lip. In other cases apparent cure can be followed by recurrent trouble at any time, as we have seen above.

The natural history of each particular cancer is clearly of paramount importance. Some grow so slowly that the patient can lead a comfortable and useful life for many years in the presence of the primary growth, even with secondaries too – e.g. some types of breast, parotid and thyroid cancers. *Ten-year* and *fifteen-year* survival figures are even more valuable than five-year survivals, but it requires an elaborate follow-up organisation to provide these. Yet it is only from painstaking statistics of this kind that we can derive sound knowledge both of the natural history of cancer and the real effects of treatment.

Survival figures are essential for estimating the success of radical treatment, but are only of limited value in assessing the effects of palliative treatment. We may be unable to achieve complete eradication or permanent control of a cancer, yet treatment may lengthen life, control primary or secondary disease even for years, alleviate painful symptoms and improve the quality of life generally. Radiotherapy, by and large, is more successful than surgery in this kind of therapy. It therefore provides a high proportion of the work of a radiotherapy department, and even apart from its success in the radical treatment of certain types of cancer, its value in palliation would amply justify the expense.

Clearly it is very difficult to be dogmatic about prognosis in cancer, even more to promise cure, and this makes for difficulty in discussion with the lay public. But we can at least be firm in our assurance that cancer is far from synonymous with 'an incurable disease'.

*Results.* If we take five-year survival as the index of success, we find the best results – i.e. an appreciable percentage of all cases surviving over five years – in cancers of the following sites:

*Five-year survival rates (all cases)*

| | | | |
|---|---|---|---|
| Skin | 75% | Uterus (cervix and body) | 45% |
| Lip | 75% | Breast | 45% |

| Testis (seminoma) | 70% | Thyroid | 40% |
| Salivary glands | 70% | Mouth | 35% |
| Larynx (vocal cords) | 50% | Bladder | 35% |

It is worth noting that many of these are included in the list of lesions for which radiation is the treatment of choice and that they are almost all *accessible* – i.e. they can be seen or felt in their early stages.

The worst results – less than 10 per cent alive at five years – are seen in:

1. Pancreas    3. Stomach    5. Leukaemia
2. Oesophagus    4. Lung    6. Hypopharynx

Other cancers occupy intermediate positions, with survival rates in the region of 20 per cent.

In discussion of results, it should always be remembered that *cancer is not one disease but many,* and each separate site represents a different disease, a different natural history and a different problem. Generalisations therefore are of very limited value. It is probably true to say that about *one cancer in three is now 'curable'* in the five-year survival sense. But this is not much help in considering an individual cancer in a particular organ, since five-year rates can range from 2 per cent to 95 per cent. In any given case the prognosis depends on many variables. These we detail in later chapters.

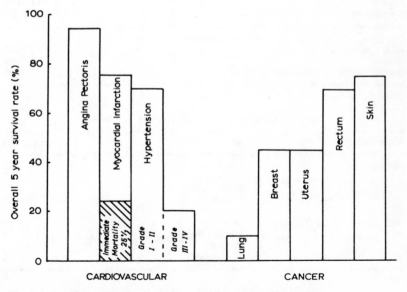

Fig. 1.4 Cardiovascular disease and cancer five-year survival rates.

At the present time the overall picture in the results of cancer treatment is not a cheerful one. Good results are obtainable in a few situations, especially for early cases of accessible growths, but in most of the common sites (e.g. lung, gastro-intestinal tract, breast, bladder, ovary) the long-term results are poor. Until the situation improves it would be wrong to be optimistic. It is improving now, albeit slowly, and will certainly improve further, perhaps much further, before the end of the century. But there is a great deal that can be done for almost all cancer patients, whether treatment is radical or palliative, and *good nursing and doctoring can make a very significant difference to the quality of life of* most of our patients. This is our best incentive and our best reward.

To help keep things in proper perspective, we may compare the prognosis in some other serious diseases.

These disorders do not rouse the same alarm and mortal fear as cancer in the public mind, yet the outlook in some cancers, as shown above, is far more favourable. These facts are important in questions of health education.

Some important data are given for reference in Tables 1.1 and 1.2.

Table 1.1 Causes of death in England and Wales – 1973
Total Population = 55 000 000)

| **All deaths** | 550 000 |
| Cardiovascular | 250 000 |
| Cancer | 113 000 |
| Respiratory | 70 000 |
| (for comparison) | |
| Motor accidents | 6500 |
| Suicide | 3600 |
| Special infections (tuberculosis, etc.) | 3000 |

Table 1.2 Commonest cancers (England and Wales)

| Males (%) | Site | Females (%) |
| --- | --- | --- |
| 30 | Lung | 5 |
| | Breast | 25 |
| 20 | Digestive tract | 20 |
| | Uterus | 10 |
| | Ovary | 5 |
| 10 | Skin | 10 |
| 7 | Urinary tract | |
| 7 | Prostate | |
| 5 | Lymphomas | 5 |

# 2. Growth and Growths: Normal and Abnormal

*What can be avoided,*
*Whose end is purpos'd by the mighty gods?*
                              Shakespeare (Julius Caesar)

Cancer is a pathological variation of normal growth.

Growth is a fundamental property of living things, and the most remarkable feature of it is the beautiful way in which it is organised and controlled from conception to maturity. Rates of growth vary greatly. Growth in the fetus is very rapid indeed – more so than in any cancer – then gradually diminishes until adulthood.

The basic unit of growth is the individual cell, beginning with the fertilised ovum. Reproduction is by cell division, and cells arise only from cells. This holds good both for initial growth and for 'wear and tear' replacement and repair.

Growth rates vary widely between different tissues. At one extreme, nerve and muscle cells are all present at birth and if later destroyed can never be replaced. At the other extreme is the bone marrow, where blood cells are in constant production. Since the red cell has a normal life of only four months, over two million red cells must be produced every second. Besides the marrow, the fastest growing tissues are the lining epithelium of the intestine (which is replaced every two days), the skin (epidermis) and the male gonad (sperm cells). In fact, about 2 per cent of our body cells die and are replaced every day. Other organs have a much lower replacement rate, for example the liver and kidney, but losses can be made good when necessary.

## Cell division (mitosis)

The mechanism of cell reproduction is the same for normal and abnormal growth and is of fundamental importance for our subject (Fig. 2.1). The whole process is governed by the nucleus of the cell. The onset of mitosis is signalled by a disturbance in the nuclear contents, which now take the shape of a tangled skein (Greek 'mitos' – thread). This next divides into a definite number of segments (46 in humans) called *chromosomes* (Greek for 'coloured bodies' as they stain darkly). Chromosomes are chains of tiny structures called *genes,* which are the physico-chemical basis of all the 'characters' of cells and therefore of the individuals they compose. ('Gene' is Greek for 'beget'. 'Kin' is from the same root.)

Next, each chromosome splits into halves which travel in opposite directions towards the poles of the cell. This ensures the same number of chromosomes in the two daughter cells. Each set of daughter chromosomes is gathered together into another tangled skein to form the nucleus of a new cell. Finally, the body of the parent cell assumes an hour-glass shape by constriction round the waist; this deepens to divide the cell into two, each with its own nucleus and full set of chromosomes and genes.

## Control and differentiation

To develop into the various organs with widely different structure and function, cells must specialise. This process is called *differentiation*. An important general consequence is that the more highly differentiated cells become, the less likely they are to divide.

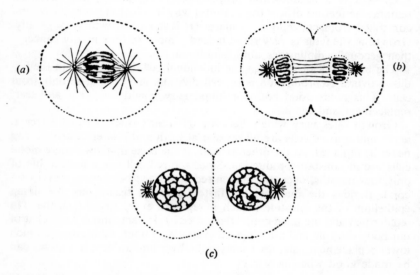

Fig. 2.1 Diagram of the essential changes taking place in cell division (mitosis). The chromosomes are seen in (a) moving towards opposite ends of the cell. In (b) the cell body is seen in process of division and the two daughter nuclei are nearly complete. In (c) the two new cells are almost completely separated, each with its own nucleus. (*Davies, 'X-ray Therapy'*)

Clearly there are delicate controlling mechanisms at work which determine the various degrees of differentiation; the size of organs and of the whole organism; the maintenance of a balance between normal destruction and regeneration. We know almost nothing about these mechanisms of control and differentiation and this ignorance bedevils our whole insight into the problems of abnormal growth, especially cancer.

*Neoplasia*

We must distinguish several varieties of abnormal growth:

a. *Hypertrophy* of organs, as in heart muscle when the heart has to work against increased resistance. Its constituent cells are enlarged and some of their nuclei may also be enlarged and bizarre.

b. *Hyperplasia* – cells are more numerous and more tightly packed with a high incidence of mitosis. It may precede cancer in epithelial surfaces and glands (e.g. endometrium, thyroid).

c. *Metaplasia* – replacement by a cell type not normally present in an organ – e.g. as a result of inflammation, transitional epithelium of the urinary tract may change to squamous and become keratinised.

d. *Neoplasia*. Neoplasm is Greek for 'new growth'. Another general term often used is 'tumour' which means simply 'swelling' and was originally used for enlargements due to injury, inflammation, cancer or anything else. The word is now usually restricted to neoplastic swellings. *Neoplasms* are in two broad classes:

1. Benign or simple.
2. Malignant or cancerous.

*Benign growths* are universal since they include the common birthmarks – everyone has a few, e.g. moles (pigmented or not), simple melanomas, papillomatous warts, fibro-fatty tags, infantile angiomas. They are harmless and usually of no more than cosmetic importance. Very rarely they may become malignant, e.g. a simple melanoma may become a malignant melanoma.

Their growth is strictly localised and never widespread, but they can be dangerous in certain situations, e.g. a simple meningioma may exert fatal pressure on the brain, whereas a similar lesion on a limb would be merely inconvenient.

*Malignant growths* are the cancers. There is no universally acceptable definition of cancer, but it has some essential behavioural qualities. *The important difference between a simple and a malignant new growth is that the latter possesses the power of 'invasion' while the former does not* (Fig. 2.2). They may grow slowly or rapidly, but if not successfully treated will lead to death sooner or later, unless death from some other cause intervenes. Growth is by local invasion at first, at the expense of surrounding tissues; later spread takes place to other parts of the body by metastasis via blood or lymphatic vessels.

Table 2.1 summarises the different characteristics.

## The nature and cause of cancer

We cannot point to any single feature to define cancer. Multiplication and growth are properties of most normal tissues, and the healing growth that repairs a cut finger is faster than that of a cancer. But such growth is under control – when the wound is healed, growth ceases. Malignant cells are under no such controlling restraint. We tend to think of a cancer as rapidly growing. In general, the cells of a cancer grow no faster than their

Table 2.1 Characteristics of neoplasms

| Benign | Malignant |
|---|---|
| Growth usually very slow, often ceases after a time. | Growth variable – may be very rapid. |
| Usually encapsulated. | Usually not encapsulated. |
| Growth by expansion. | Growth by infiltration. |
| Remain localised. | Metastasise (lymph or blood etc.). |
| Histological appearance similar to normal tissue. | Histology diverges more or less from the normal, but often widely. |
| Little or no destruction of normal tissue. | Tissue destruction eventually extensive if untreated. |
| Not fatal (except from mechanical pressure in special sites). | Always eventually fatal if not halted in time. |

normal counterparts, and in fact often more slowly. But all normal cell growth is under control, and addition of new cells is matched by loss of old cells, in accordance with the physiological needs of the organ. In a cancer these balancing constraints are lost, new cells pile up regardless of physiological need, and thus *appear* to be growing rapidly.

What has happened when a normal cell starts to behave as a malignant cell? It is tempting to suppose it has acquired some new property, a mysterious faculty for unlimited growth. The truth seems to be that it has not gained anything at all, but has lost something. All cells possess – or in their developmental history once possessed – theoretically unlimited growth potential, but this is subordinated to the controlling process – of unknown nature – responsible for tissue organisation. The cancer cell has lost the capacity to respond to normal control mechanisms – it is a delinquent, unresponsive to civilising influences. It is easier to lose something than to acquire something – it is relatively easy for a normal cell to become cancerous but virtually impossible for a cancer cell to become normal. It follows that treatment must aim at the destruction of every cancer cell, or failing that, the abolition of their capacity to reproduce. Otherwise residual cells will survive to form recurrent growths.

## Irritation

If we paint a patch of skin in a mouse or rabbit repeatedly with tar, a skin cancer (epithelioma) can eventually be produced. The particular chemical compound responsible has been isolated and many other similar carcinogens (i.e. 'cancer-producers') are known. Their mode of action is still obscure, but it is at least interesting to note that many compounds, including hormones, which occur naturally in the human body have related chemical structures.

This type of chemical *carcinogenesis* occurs in man, e.g. long years of work with tar are liable to produce skin cancers on exposed hands and faces. In 1775 Percival Pott described chimney sweep's cancer –

epithelioma of the scrotum, due to contamination with soot. There are many other industrial examples, e.g. mule-spinner's cancer from the oil used in treating yarn in spinning mills, and similar lesions from lubricating oils in machine tools. Internal cancers can also arise from chemical substances, e.g. workers in the dye and rubber industries excrete compounds in the urine which are liable to cause bladder cancer. The most important example of all is the production of lung cancer by tobacco smoke. It is also possible that inhaled tobacco products excreted in the urine contribute significantly to bladder cancer, which is on the increase.

In all these instances, there seems to be a common factor of chronic irritation at work. We cannot pin-point the mechanism – all we can say is that it is a reaction to injurious agents, a constantly repeated cycle of insult and repair until the reparative processes become 'fatigued' and control of growth is lost. The result is a cancer, with production of changed cells often of peculiar shape and size and with a capacity for rapid and purposeless multiplication with no regard to either the local or the general economy of the body. However, it is not just a matter of simple irritation in the mechanical sense. There is no correlation between the mechanically irritative and the carcinogenic properties of materials. Coal dust is highly irritant mechanically but never produces cancer; whereas soot (from coal after combustion) is a powerful carcinogen. It is a *chemical* factor in the products of combustion that is the responsible agent.

Another important type of irritant factor is *radiation,* e.g. ultra-violet rays, invisible components of sunlight, responsible for suntan can cause skin cancer after prolonged exposure – as in farm workers and sailors, and in sun-blessed countries like Australia, Argentina or southern U.S.A.

### X-rays

Before the dangers of radiation were appreciated, many pioneer workers developed skin cancers, especially on the fingers. Other carcinogenic effects included leukaemia, and diagnostic radiology is a further potential source of danger (see p. 110) especially where growing tissue is involved. For example, some childhood cancers including leukaemia, are thought to be due to pelvic radiography of the mother during pregnancy.

### Radioactive mineral ores

Workers at certain mines in Bohemia – where Marie Curie obtained the pitchblende from which she isolated radium – were for centuries susceptible to 'Mine Disease', now recognised to have been lung cancer. The atmosphere in the mines contained radon (see p. 54) and its various decay products were deposited in the lungs, giving off beta and gamma rays and the even more dangerous (since they are more intensely ionising) alpha particles (see Ch. 4). The average induction period was about 20 years.

Comparable effects resulted from luminous paint for watch dials, among the girls in a factory in New Jersey (U.S.A.). The paint contained small amounts of radioactive material (including radium) and when the workers pointed the brushes between their lips, traces of paint were ingested, absorbed and deposited mainly in bone where they continued to emit alphas, betas and gammas. Some died in a few years from aplastic anaemia; others developed bone sarcomas after some fifteen years. Similar bone cancers have resulted from regular drinking of radioactive spa waters.

*Atomic bombs* offer a striking example. The survivors at Hiroshima and Nagasaki suffered an increased incidence of cancer, especially leukaemia. This is an effect of acute rather than chronic irritation on the highly susceptible bone marrow which is normally the site of rapid cell proliferation. A clinically important case is the production of leukaemia (as well as other cancers) after X-ray treatment to large areas of the spine for ankylosing spondylitis. These examples are enough to show why we are increasingly reluctant nowadays to use ionising radiation in treatment of non-malignant conditions.

*Infection*

The role of chronic infection is hard to isolate but it is probably an important factor in cancer production in e.g. the mouth, and also the cervix. In both these instances cancer is commoner as we descend the social scale and seems to be associated with poor personal hygiene.

*Hormones*

We have already mentioned the chemical resemblance of hormones to some known carcinogens. A milestone in experimental cancer research was passed when administration of natural ovarian hormone was shown to produce breast cancers in mice. This at once opened up the possibility of physiological substances acting in the body as carcinogens, though the amounts of hormone needed experimentally were relatively huge and there may be no real parallel with natural events in humans.

However, it is reasonable to postulate hormonal influences in breast cancer. The breast is an unstable organ, wirth cyclical growth changes, subsidence and regeneration, depending on a delicate balance of endocrine secretions. There is good reason to believe that abnormalities of hormone patterns – i.e. of growth stimulus – may be common factors in initiating breast cancer (see p. 111) and this also applies to other organs subject to hormonal influences, e.g. testis, uterus, ovary, thyroid, even kidney (see Ch. 12).

*Worms and cancer*

There are several examples in animals of cancers caused by worm infestation. In some parts of the world notably Egypt there is good reason to believe that bilharziasis is the external irritant factor responsible for the high incidence of bladder cancer (see p. 153).

*Viruses and cancer*

Viruses can unquestionably induce cancer in animals and also in plants — e.g. leukaemia in mice, sarcoma in chickens, skin tumours in rabbits, even breast cancer in mice. An immense amount of laboratory work has been done in this field and the virus theory of cancer has enjoyed great popularity and still does. It obviously links up with immunological aspects discussed below. One speculative hypothesis is that there is a widespread virus lurking in human cells, normally harmless, but capable of malignant activation by various stimuli (physical, chemical, radiation, etc.).

It seems reasonable enough to think that at least some human cancers are due to virus infection, but it remains true that so far there is no definite proof of this for any cancer in man.

*Resistance to cancer: Immunology*

*Antigen and antibody. Anti* is Latin for 'against', 'opposed to'; 'gen' is Greek for 'producing'. Antigen is something that produces an opponent. Anything 'foreign' to the body, is liable to provoke the production of opposing chemical substance called 'antibody' to neutralise it. The stimulant (bacterium, virus, vaccine etc.) is the antigen, the opponent produced (by the reticulo-endothelial system) is the antibody.

In the nature of things, normal cells are not antigenic (otherwise they would not be normal!) but abnormal cells may be. Since many millions of cells are dividing by mitosis in the body every day, mutation, though rare, must occasionally occur and produce abnormal cells with some degree of antigenicity. These abnormal cells are likely to be promptly attacked and destroyed by lymphocytes etc. which are the body's 'watchdogs.'

Resistance to infection (by antibodies etc.) is well recognised. The possibility of a viral origin of cancer raises comparable possibilities of antigens, antibodies and antisera in treatment — but these are as yet little more than theoretical.

However, some form of resistance to cancer does appear to exist, and to play a real part in determining whether a cancer arises or not. It is even possible that the normal body is constantly producing microscopic cancers which are prevented from developing by existing defence mechanisms, just as bacteria and viruses are constantly antagonised and neutralised by the reticulo-endothelial system before clinical infection can occur.

We know that many clinical cancers continually shed cancer cells into the blood stream and they can readily be detected in the venous outflow at the time of surgical resection. But only a small proportion of these give rise to metastases — the cancer cells are presumably killed or incapacitated before they can 'take' at any site. Another suggestive feature is the local infiltration round some cancers by lymphocytes and plasma cells which are components of the lymphoreticular system. We know, for example, that breast cancers which have this infiltration carry a better prognosis than those which do not.

Immunological factors therefore appear to be important both in the rise and spread of cancer. There have been many reported instances of tumour regression after injections of vaccines or other foreign material. The mechanism is obscure − possibly it may trigger the body's immune defence system into treating the tumour as foreign tissue and rejecting it in the same way as a transplant. Vaccine is now proving useful in the treatment of some leukaemias (p. 183). Immune mechanisms seem to be the major factors in the control of choriocarcinoma (p. 233) and Burkitt's lymphoma (p. 234).

Whether the immunological front will achieve worthwhile success in the campaign against cancer still remains to be seen.

## Heredity in cancer

'Can cancer be inherited?' is a question commonly and anxiously asked by patients and relations. The short answer is − No.

We can in-breed mice so that they all develop cancer but this laboratory experiment has no possible counterpart in humans. This is not to say that inherited − i.e. genetic − factors have no importance. They undoubtedly have, but they are only one set of factors among many and to determine a cancer there must be a combination of factors at work − cancer is multi-factorial. Hereditary factors may decide which particular organ is liable to develop cancer and there are certainly some families where several members develop e.g. breast cancer. But the cancer itself is not inherited, though the predisposition may be and other factors must be operative before the cancer can arise.

Further evidence comes from identical twins who develop cancers. If heredity is important, we would expect them to develop similar cancers at about the same time, but this is very uncommon (though commoner than in non-identical twins). Hereditary factors do have some importance here, but as usual environmental factors seem to be far more important than genetic.

However, there are two genuine examples of genetically determined cancers:

a. retinoblastoma − a rare cancer affecting the eyes of infants and often found in several children of the same parents or in parent and child. This is the only instance where the growth is malignant from the start.

b. familial multiple polyposis of colon − where the polyps, originally benign, later become malignant.

## Infectivity of cancer

'Is cancer catching?' is another frequent question. 'Is there any danger to the children in the house?' There is no evidence whatever that cancer can be caught in this way − there is not a single recorded instance − and complete reassurance can be given.

Even if a virus is ever proved to be involved in human cancer it is unlikely that this statement will need changing for practical purposes.

## Injury and cancer

It is popularly believed that physical trauma may cause cancer and a patient may attribute say a breast tumour to a blow received previously. This belief may lead to claims for compensation if the injury was received at work. It is extremely unlikely that trauma alone can later produce a cancer, but it may draw attention to a tumour previously unnoticed.

The incidence of injury is so very high and the cases where even a moderately plausible case for a cause and effect association with cancer can be made out are so very few, that it is best to conclude that no definite relationship exists.

Chronic injury, e.g. from asbestos dust in the lungs − or tobacco smoke! − falls of course in a different category (see above).

## The natural history of cancer

It seems wiser not to speak of 'The Cause' of cancer but of multiple causes or causative factors. Though one factor may be the 'last straw', it is probable that in nearly all cases there must be a combination of causative factors at work, including genetic, hormonal, metabolic, inflammatory, physical, chemical, thermal, and environmental generally.

## The earliest stage of malignancy

This is clearly a subject of fundamental importance since it is the stage where we can hope for complete eradication. In recent years some progress has been made in recognising these early changes in epithelial surfaces.

Pre-cancerous lesions may be recognised, a halfway house between the normal and the frankly malignant. Individual cells are abnormal, but the picture of invasive cancer is not present and the term *'pre-invasive cancer'* is sometimes used. In such cases experience shows that malignancy is very likely to follow, though it may be many years later.

Examples of pre-cancerous lesions are:

a. Hyperkeratosis of skin − small warty growths: may be due to chronic irritation by tar, sunlight, X-rays etc.
b. Leucoplakia − thickened whitish patches on mucosal surfaces especially in the mouth.
c. Papilloma of bladder − commonly multiple (papillomatosis).
d. Polyp of the bowel − including rectum.
e. Stage 0 of carcinoma of cervix − see pp. 35 and 124.
f. Plummer − Vinson syndrome in post-cricoid cancer (p. 142).
g. Paget's disease of bone (p. 168).
h. Congenitally abnormal organs, e.g. imperfectly descended testis.

Although cancer may possibly arise from a change in a single cell, it is normally due to a 'field' change in a whole area. It is not surprising to find that many foci may be abnormal in a tissue where cancer has arisen, either naked eye or microscopically. The same factors responsible for a clinical cancer will often produce changes in the rest of the organ, e.g. multiple malignant or pre-malignant patches may be present in a breast removed for cancer. In other words the whole epithelium may be unstable and liable to degenerate into malignancy at multiple points. Thus a patient treated for cancer of the lip may later develop one on the tongue, then on the buccal cheek, then in the pharynx . . .

## The spread of cancer

Growth may be (a) continuous, by local enlargement of the *primary* mass, or (b) discontinuous, by *secondary* growth elsewhere, near or far, with normal tissue intervening – this is called *Metastasis*. Spread may occur in several ways:

1. Local invasion
2. By lymphatic vessels
3. By blood vessels
4. Across cavities

### 1. Local invasion

Multiplication of cells results in a microscopic mass which will enlarge to become visible or palpable or produce other clinical effects. Cancer cells insinuate themselves between the normal cells and compete for the available nourishment. Normal tissue will eventually be disorganised and destroyed, depending on the blood supply and the available 'elbow room'.

The edge of the tumour is therefore ill-defined (Fig. 2.2) and complete excision by surgery correspondingly difficult and uncertain. A generous margin of apparently normal tissue should always be removed, but even then microscopic examination – or the later clinical course – may show that some malignant cells have been left behind. If so, they will eventually produce a *local recurrence* if nothing further is done.

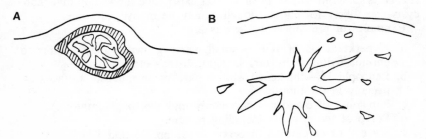

Fig. 2.2 Showing the difference between a benign tumour (A) contained by a definite capsule and a malignant tumour (B) actively invading the tumour bed.

Ulceration on a surface internal or external may cause bleeding and secondary infection. Erosion of a large vessel may cause serious even fatal haemorrhage. Cancer cells may be temporarily halted at a barrier, e.g. bone, but even this will be invaded and eroded.

Functional changes may follow. For instance, a growth in the oesophagus or bowel may cause obstruction, damage to the brain may cause headaches or fits, involvement of the liver or obstruction of the bile duct may lead to jaundice and liver failure, just as spread of cancer of the cervix to the ureters may result in renal failure and uraemia. Unless they can be relieved by treatment (usually surgery or radiation) these changes are liable to be fatal, even in the absence of metastases.

Pain will occur when nerve endings are involved but (contrary to popular belief) it is a late symptom, often very late.

### 2. Lymphatic spread

At some stage of a cancer's development, local lymphatic capillaries may be involved and isolated cells or clumps of cells may be carried in the lymph flow to one or more of the regional lymph nodes. (They are still often called 'glands', a misnomer from the days when they were thought to be organs of secretion. It is time the old name was abandoned.)

If the cancer cells survive and multiply in the node, they form a secondary deposit or *metastasis* and the node may eventually become palpably enlarged, e.g. secondary axillary nodes in breast cancer. From one node, further deposits may arise in other nodes along the chain, e.g. spread to supraclavicular nodes may come from internal mammary or axillary nodes (Fig. 8.2, p. 113).

From lymphatic vessels and nodes cancer cells may eventually enter the general blood circulation, just as lymph itself does.

### 3. Blood spread

Cancer cells enter the blood stream commonly from the region of the primary growth by direct invasion of blood capillaries or via lymphatics. Metastatic growth can arise in almost any site in the body, but there is a definite preference for certain organs − after regional nodes, the commonest are liver, lungs and bone.

*Metastasis is the chief danger in any cancer* and the cause of death in most of the fatal cases, from gross involvement of vital organs.

In general, carcinoma shows a marked tendency to early lymphatic spread, whereas sarcoma usually spreads via the blood stream.

A secondary deposit may give the first clinical evidence of cancer. For example, a tiny primary in the nasopharynx may give rise to much larger secondary nodes in the neck or a supraclavicular node may be the first evidence of a pancreatic growth. Pain from bone secondaries − or even a pathological fracture − may be the presenting feature in lung or breast cancer. In some cases secondaries may dominate the picture from the start, and the primary may be so small and insignificant that it is not discovered till post-mortem examination (or not even then!).

### 4. Cavity spread

a. Cancer cells in the upper abdomen, e.g. from a gastric cancer — may be dislodged into the peritoneal cavity and come to rest in the ovary or pouch of Douglas where they will form a secondary deposit. Similarly an ovarian cancer in the pelvis may deposit seedlings on peritoneal or mesenteric surfaces.

b. A similar sequence may occur in the thorax, from one part of the pleural surface to another.

c. Cells from an intracranial growth, e.g. medulloblastoma of cerebellum — may be seeded into the cerebrospinal fluid and form deposits on other brain surfaces or in the spinal canal.

d. Cells from the upper urinary tract, e.g. renal pelvis — may be carried down in the urine to form a deposit in ureter or bladder.

As the word 'malignant' implies, death is the natural result of un-treated — or unsuccessfully treated — cancer. It occurs from general exhaustion, liver or kidney failure, haemorrhage, terminal broncho-pneumonia, cerebral complications etc. Cancer's grim reputation then has a realistic basis and though the overtones of the word are today less horrific than they were in former generations, they are still sombre enough to prevent our challenging the use of the adjective 'malignant' — at least yet.

## Growth rate of cancers

Theoretically a cancer could start as a single abnormal cell, which divides to form two cells, then four cells, then eight cells . . . and so on. And the same could occur with a single celled metastasis. Single cells can produce cancers in laboratory animals, but under human conditions it is far more likely that numbers of cells in foci become changed under some carcinogenic stimulus and it would hardly be worth arguing whether one or more cells were the true originators of the clinical cancer.

It is important to distinguish between *histological* cancer and *clinical* cancer. At the earliest recognisable stage, abnormal cells may be detected under the microscope, e.g. by abnormal staining or abnormal shape of the nucleus. This is the basis of the cytological detection of early or pre-invasive cancer of the cervix (p. 35). At a later stage cellular abnormalities — abnormal shapes and sizes of cells, bizarre nuclei etc. — and early local invasion would be found microscopically, though there might be no clinical evidence whatever — no tumour, no ulcer, no symptoms. In the earliest stages of cancer the histological diagnosis may be very difficult, for there is no sharp boundary between the normal and the pathological and two equally expert pathologists may disagree whether or not a cellular hyperplasia is malignant. Such doubt is common for instance after examining prostates removed for urinary obstruction or thyroids removed for nodular goitre.

There will thus always be a latent interval from the inception of a cancer to its first histologically recognisable state and a still longer interval before its first clinical sign – visible tumour, ulceration, bleeding etc. Clearly these intervals are matters of life and death, and the more rapid the growth, the shorter the latent interval.

It is instructive to consider these intervals in concrete terms (Figs. 2.3, 2.4). If a typical human cancer cell divides after a certain time – so many hours or days to become two cells, the *doubling time* – and if the daughter cells keep up regular division in the same way, then simple calculation shows that it will take 20 doublings to produce a mass one cubic millimetre containing one million cells. This is about the smallest tumour mass one could ever hope to detect clinically. After 10 further doublings – i.e. 30 in all – there would be a mass of one cubic centimetre weighing one gram, containing about 1000 million cells. This would generally be considered an early lesion and we might well congratulate ourselves if we picked up, say, a breast cancer as small as this.

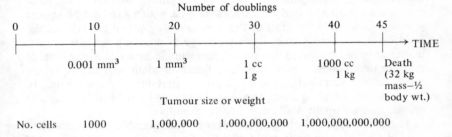

Fig. 2.3 Tumour growth by successive cell doublings (see text).

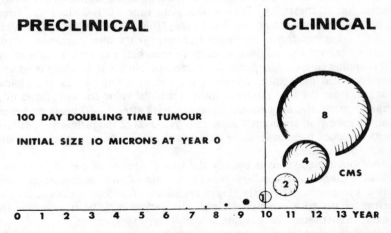

Fig 2.4 Growth of tumour with a doubling time of 100 days. Note the long pre-clinical interval from inception to diagnosis. A clinical tumour can easily be ten years old when first detected.

Ten more doubling times, i.e. 40 in all – would bring the mass to one kilogram, by which time of course there would be gross clinical changes, maybe even cachexia. If a patient could possibly survive five more doubling times, i.e. 45 in all – it would mean a mass of 30 kilograms or half the body weight – an unlikely event, but certainly fatal.

But let us note that the time for 30 doublings, i.e. from one cell to one gram – is at least twice the length of time from one gram to death. When we reflect that a cancer can rarely be diagnosed before the stage of one gram (= one cubic centimetre), it is clear that the greater part of its lifetime will already be behind it at the time of diagnosis, in fact about two-thirds of its total history, with all that this implies in terms of metastasis. The clinical period is therefore only the visible tip of a pre-clinical 'iceberg'.

These calculations are theoretical and may even seem fanciful at first, but there is good reason to believe that they are not far from the truth. Evidence from both animals and human cancers suggests that most tumours do grow at a fairly constant rate – i.e. with a fixed doubling time – which varies little for most of the tumour's life. Actual growth will depend on this doubling time. Our knowledge of doubling times is scanty, but it has been possible to measure it, for example by serial X-ray films of primary or secondary masses in lung fields, or mammograms of breast tumours. Not surprisingly there is a great variability in growth rates. In lung cancers, doubling times were found to range from 11 to 164 days, in breast cancers up to 450 days, i.e. 15 months.

These figures are of obvious importance. For example, with a doubling time of 60 days a tumour could take five years to grow to a diagnosable mass of one gram – and this is about the diagnostic boundary for a lung cancer on a chest film. With a doubling time of 100 days the pre-diagnostic interval would last 8-10 years (Fig. 2.4). They would also explain how secondaries can appear many years after removal of the primary growth. As we have seen, more than half a tumour's life – about 30 doubling times – has generally passed before it can be diagnosed and removed and metastases could be shed at any stage in its pre-clinical history, from the first doubling to the thirtieth. With doubling times of a year or more, the appearance of secondaries after 20-30 years and even longer, following apparently successful removal of the primary – and this certainly does happen in some cases, especially in breast cancer – could easily be explained.

Although metastasis is usually the tragic element in cancer, it is only the final stages of secondary growth that are of clinical importance and cause symptoms. The early stages are silent. If we can reduce a growth or metastasis to a sub-clinical level, the patient may be trouble-free for years, even though harbouring a silently growing lesion.

It follows that 'cure' in the popular sense is not the only – not even the best – measure of success in cancer therapy.

## Spontaneous regression of cancer

This sounds like a contradiction in terms, but it does seem possible that cancer can disappear spontaneously, that is without obvious treatment. We are rightly sceptical of all such claims and demand convincing proof, including expert histological confirmation. There are several hundred articles in medical journals describing alleged cases, and one whole book reviewing the subject and accepting the claim in some 180 cases.

As an example, there is a small series of bladder tumours confirmed as malignant in the usual way by biopsy. Urinary diversion was carried out by ureteric transplantation as a preliminary measure, and after a suitable interval the bladder was removed at cystectomy. Examination of the resected bladders showed no remaining cancer tissue. Presumably there had been a carcinogenic stimulus probably a chemical factor in the urine acting on the bladder epithelium. When this stimulus was removed by urinary diversion, the epithelium was able to recover its integrity. If this is really so, then it does appear possible that the earliest stages of carcinogenesis may sometimes be reversible and underlines the possibility of *resistance* to cancer.

Over half of the collected cases occurred in four types of cancer-carcinoma of kidney (hypernephroma), neuroblastoma, malignant melanoma and choriocarcinoma. In renal cancer and maligant melanoma, *hormonal* influences are known to be concerned and it seems certain that they must have played some part in the process. Choriocarcinoma (p. 232) is a peculiar kind of cancer of different behaviour from most cancers and it is highly probable that *immunological* reactions are involved in its regression. In neuroblastoma (p. 239) spontaneous maturation into the simple adult type of ganglioneuroma is known to occur in a small proportion of cases, about 1 per cent.

In other cases, bacterial infection seems to have played a part and possibly the antigen-antibody mechanism may have been responsible. Many years ago bacterial toxins were actually used in cancer therapy and seemed to be helpful at times. The present day revival of interest in the immunology of cancer (see above) makes these cases particularly interesting.

The total number of these cases is relatively very small, so small that they might seem practically speaking unimportant. However the significance of these cases lies in the support they lend to the concept of biological controls even in cancer, and in reinforcing the hope that future research may yet give us better methods than surgery, radiation and poison, which are after all the very crude instruments we have at present.

## Classification of neoplasms

Table 2.2 lists the chief types. The ending 'oma' is used to indicate a neoplasm, just as 'itis' indicates inflammation. It took many centuries for the concept of cancer as a distinctive entity to evolve. The suffix 'oma'

Table 2.2 Types of neoplasms

| Benign | Tissue of origin | Malignant |
|---|---|---|
| | **Epithelium** = surface tissue | General name = **Carcinoma** |
| Papilloma | Squamous epithelium | Squamous carcinoma or epithelioma |
| | Transitional cell epithelium | Transitional cell carcinoma |
| | Basal cells of epidermis | Basal cell carcinoma or Rodent ulcer |
| Adenoma | Glandular epithelium | Adenocarcinoma |
| | **Supporting tissues** | General name = **Sarcoma** |
| Fibroma | Fibrous tissue | Fibrosarcoma |
| Myoma | Muscle | Myosarcoma |
| Leiomyoma | Smooth muscle | Leiomyosarcoma |
| Rhabdomyoma | Striated muscle | Rhabdomyosarcoma |
| Lipoma | Fat | Liposarcoma |
| Chondroma | Cartilage | Chondrosarcoma |
| Osteoma | Bone | Osteosarcoma (osteogenic sarcoma) |
| Synovioma | Synovial membrane | Synovial sarcoma |
| | **Lympho-Reticular tissue** | General name = **Reticulosis** or *Malignant Lymphoma* |
| Lymphoma | Lymphoid tissue – including spleen | Lymphosarcoma Reticulum cell (histiocytic) sarcoma Hodgkin's disease |
| | In skin | Mycosis fungoides |
| | Blood forming tissues: – white cells | Leukaemia (myeloid, lymphatic) |
| | – red cells | Polycythaemia Rubra Vera |
| Solitary Myeloma | Plasma cell | Multiple myeloma (myelomatosis) |
| | **Pigment cells** | |
| Mole or naevus (benign melanoma) | Skin Mucosa Eye (choroid) | Malignant Melanoma (melanocarcinoma, melanosarcoma) |
| (Haem) angioma | **Blood vessels** | (Haem) angiosarcoma |

| Benign | Tissue of Origin | Malignant |
|--------|------------------|-----------|
| | **Intracranial** | |
| | Supporting tissue of central nervous system | Glioma (this includes astrocytoma, glioblastoma, oligodendroglioma ependymoma, pinealoma etc.) |
| Meningioma | Meninges | |
| Pituitary Adenoma (chromophobe, eosinophil, basophil) | Pituitary gland | |
| Hydatidiform Mole | **Placenta** (fetal tissue) | Chorionepithelioma (Choriocarcinoma) |
| Dermoid Cyst | **Gonad** | Teratoma |
| Benign Teratoma | (germ cells) | Seminoma (male) Dysgerminoma (female) |
| | **In children** Kidney | Nephroblastoma (= Wilms's tumour or embryoma) |
| | Sympathetic nerve tissue | Neuroblastoma |
| | Cerebellum | Medulloblastoma |
| | Retina | Retinoblastoma |

N.B. This table is not complete. For rarer types, standard works on pathology should be consulted.

was applied to swellings of any nature. This relic of the past survives to-day in the use of names like tuberculoma, haematoma, etc.

Malignant neoplasms are *cancers*. Cancer is Latin for 'crab' and a picture of a crab is often used to symbolise cancer. The ancients used this name because swollen veins are often seen radiating from advanced growths, giving a picture resembling a crab's limbs.

Most cancers are in one of these sub-divisions:

### 1. Carcinoma        2. Sarcoma        3. Reticulosis

*Carcinoma* is from the Greek for 'crab' but it is used in a more restricted sense than cancer and applied to malignancy arising in surface (i.e. epithelial) tissues. This is the largest and most important group of cancers — in fact 75 per cent of all cancers are carcinomas.

*Squamous epithelium* (squamous is Latin for 'scaly', from the microscopic appearance resembling fishscales) lines the skin – where it is called epidermis – and the mucosal surfaces of oral and nasal cavities, accessory sinuses, pharynx, most of oesophagus, respiratory tract (larynx, trachea, bronchi) middle ear, vagina, cervix. The terms squamous carcinoma, squamous epithelioma, and simply epithelioma are used synonymously.

*Glandular (secretory) epithelium* may form a naked eye surface (as in the bowel) or remain microscopic (as in the breast). In the case of the latter it is continuous with an ordinary surface from which it is derived by a complicated downfolding process, the proximal part of which forms the duct (Fig. 2.5). The ductless endocrine glands lose their original ducts and their secretions pass into the blood stream.

A            B

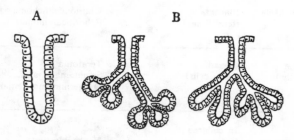

Fig. 2.5 Diagrams of simple and complex glands, showing their formation by infolding and down-growths of surface layers. The terminal parts become the secreting cells (e.g. milk-secreting cells of breast and the initial parts form the main ducts along which the secretion passes. (*Whillis, Elementary Anatomy and Physiology, Churchill*)

This type of epithelium lines the whole of the alimentary tract from lower oesophagus to upper part of anal canal as well as all the glands opening into it including pancreas and liver. It also lines the sebaceous and sweat glands of the skin, the endometrium and mammary gland, the salivary and mucous glands of respiratory and upper digestive tract (including mouth and nose), the kidney, ovary and testis and all endocrine glands (pituitary, thyroid, parathyroid, suprarenal).

*Adenocarcinomas* (Greek 'aden' = gland) may retain some of the secretory function of the parent tissue, e.g. mucoid secretion in nasal cavity, hormonal secretion in thyroid. Cyst formation is common, e.g. thyroid, ovary (called cystadenoma and cystadenocarcinoma). Spread from carcinoma is commonly to regional lymph nodes and also via the blood to lungs, liver, brain etc.

*Sarcoma* is from the Greek for 'flesh' after the fleshy appearance of many of these tumours. The commonest is the fibrosarcoma in the thigh or buttock. Spread of sarcoma is usually blood-borne to lungs and rarely to lymph nodes.

*Gliomas* (Glia is Greek for 'glue') arise from the specialised connective tissue of the central nervous system (brain and spinal cord).

*Reticulosis* (Latin reticulum = 'network'). The reticulo-endothelial system is a widespread group which includes the blood-forming bone marrow, the lymph nodes, spleen, and parts of the liver and thymus. The group of reticuloses is a very mixed one, of variable malignancy, ranging from the semi-benign polycythaemia to the rapidly fatal acute leukaemia. They may arise at many foci simultaneously or spread successively from node to node − it is often difficult to be sure.

## Staging of cancers

It is of the greatest practical importance to estimate the geographical extent of spread of any tumour. We call this:

*Staging*

There are various criteria and systems in use, but in general something like the following is adopted:

*Stage 1.* Tumour confined to organ of origin.

*Stage 2.* Local lymph nodes invaded.

*Stage 3.* Distant nodes invaded, or local spread beyond organ of origin.

*Stage 4.* Blood-borne metastases present.

Staging is based on the *clinical* findings (including radiological) before treatment is begun and is therefore not necessarily the same as the *pathological* staging based on histological examination. Staging enables us to group our cases and to make meaningful comparisons with cases at other centres.

The best example of staging is in carcinoma of cervix. This has been internationally accepted so that results of treatment all over the world can be profitably compared. Details are given on p. 124. Breast cancer also lends itself to staging (see p. 112), but unfortunately there is so far no widely accepted international system. Another example is Hodgkin's disease (see p. 177).

*TNM system.* This is a system of staging proposed for international use and it will certainly be widely accepted before long.

**T** refers to local extension of primary **Tumour;**

**N** refers to the condition of regional lymph **Nodes;**

**M** refers to the presence of **Metastases,** beyond regional nodes.

T1 means a relatively small primary, confined to the organ of origin;

T2 means a relatively large primary, limited to the organ of origin;

T3 means infiltration of neighbouring structures;

T4 means wide involvement of neighbouring structures.

N0 − no nodes palpable;

N1 − movable nodes on same side as primary tumour.

   N1 may be further sub-divided:

   N1a − nodes not considered to contain growth;

   N1b − nodes considered to contain growth.

N2 — movable nodes on opposite side similarly subdivided into N2a and N2b.

N3 — fixed nodes.

(The system is modified in some sites where nodes cannot be examined clinically.)

M0 — no evidence of distant metastases.

M1 — distant metastases present.

Thus a very early cancer would be labelled **T1N0M0** and a very late one **T4N3M1**.

## Histological grading: differentiation

In tumour histology we are concerned not only to recognise in which organ a growth orginates, but also to assess the degree of malignancy of the constituent cells, by studying the individual cells and noting how far they diverge from the normal for that particular tissue.

Development from the embryonic and primitive to the adult and specialised is called *differentiation* and the microscopic appearance of an embryonic undifferentiated cell differs from that of a mature differentiated cell. Malignant growths may or may not grow faster than normal tissue — in fact they often do not — but they generally contain a relatively high proportion of undifferentiated cells more concerned with growth and less with function. The malignancy of a tumour in fact, is shown by the relative proportion of poorly differentiated to well differentiated cells.

Histological grading has its uses, but is not nearly as important as Staging. We define three grades:

1. well differentiated
2. poorly differentiated
3. undifferentiated — also called *anaplasic* (Greek for 'forming anew').

The more undifferentiated or anaplastic a growth appears, the more liable it is to throw off early metastases, and the worse therefore is the prognosis. On the other hand, it is likely to be more radiosensitive. Knowledge of the grading of a tumour can be one factor in deciding the best treatment of a case, and this is another reason for taking a biopsy. For example, anaplasia may well be a point against surgery and in favour of radiation, since anaplasic growths are more liable to recur locally and to have silent metastases.

However, grading has its limitations. The degree of differentiation may not be the same in all parts of a tumour, and may not be the same in metastases as in the primary. The organ involved is of more importance than the grading, e.g. a Grade 1 (well differentiated) cancer of the skin has an excellent prognosis, but the same grade in the lung has a very poor prognosis.

# 3. Public Health Aspects of Cancer

*The trouble with people is not that they don't know,*
*but that they know so much that ain't so.*
                                        Henry Wheeler Shaw (1818-1885)

### Epidemiology of cancer

Cancer affects men of all races, all colours and all countries. It affects animals too, and even plants. The study of its incidence in space and time, its variations from country to country, between different races, in different circumstances of nutrition, hygiene, employment and all kinds of environmental factors, is the province of the epidemiologist and statistician. It was this kind of study that drew attention to the important association between smoking and lung cancer.

*Cancer statistics and registration.* It is clearly of prime importance to secure full and accurate figures in all cancer cases, with details of treatment and cause of death (which may or may not be cancer). This is true of all types of disease, but particularly cancer. Using these figures as a basis, we can extract the facts about its incidence at different sites; about variations in different parts of the country and between different social classes; the effects of treatment, length of survival etc. The Registrar-General in England publishes some of these details in his annual reports. Regional Health Authorities also have cancer registers, and hospital treatment centres such as radiotherapy departments maintain their own records.

It is impossible to obtain complete coverage, for some cancers are never even reported and death certificates are by no means always reliable. But the figures are now good enough for most comparative purposes.

It is evident why we take such trouble to follow-up our cancer patients, for only from full and detailed statistics and comparisons can we assess the results of various methods of treatment – or lack of treatment.

*Age.* No age group is exempt. Cancers in childhood form a rather special group (see Ch. 14), but most cancers take many years to produce clinical symptoms. It is therefore not surprising to find an increased incidence in the older age groups. The longer we live, the greater the chance of developing cancer.

If cancer is on the increase, as it is in most countries, this is largely a reflection of the fact that people are living longer. This in turn is a tribute

to the effectiveness of public health measures – nutrition, hygiene, housing, factory inspection etc. – rather than an indictment of the health
professions.

Some two centuries ago the average expectation of life of a new-born
infant was about 30 years in Britain. Today it is about 70, and old-age
pensioners are even becoming a 'problem' in western countries. But it is
still in the 30's in many parts of the world – Africa, India, South America
etc. Even in the 19th century serious epidemics of cholera and typhoid
occurred in England and it is this type of infection, as well as the parasitic
diseases, both helped by malnutrition, which are still largely responsible
for death in the less prosperous countries. There death rates will be high,
but cancer incidence low since potential victims will be killed off before
cancer can develop.

*Geographical, racial and environmental factors*

Here are a few random findings:

1. Cancer of the stomach is rare in Indonesia (1 per cent of all cancer
deaths) but very common in Japan (50 per cent).

2. Chinese are very susceptible to cancer of naso-pharynx.

3. Liver cancer is common in Africa but uncommon elsewhere.

4. Lung cancer is uncommon in Finland and Iceland, but common in
England.

5. Cancer of cervix is very uncommon in Jewesses, and even rarer in
nuns.

6. Cancer of penis never occurs in men circumcised in infancy.

7. Breast cancer is common in the West, uncommon in Japan.

Facts like these point forcefully to the determining or at least contributory influence of various internal (including genetic and hormonal)
and external factors – for example, food deficiencies, special infections,
marriage and weaning customs, chemicals in the soil, smoking habits etc.
The epidemiologist tries to disentangle and pin-point possible factors by
comparing and contrasting different groups in different settings. It is
fascinating but difficult work beset by pitfalls. In establishing cor-
relations, it is easy to confuse cause with effect. It does not follow, for example, that because there is a higher concentration of nurses in towns
than in villages, the higher incidence of cancer in towns is somehow due
to the nurses! Perhaps the greatest triumph in this field has come from
the prolonged patient statistical work which finally removed all doubt
about the cause-and-effect association between smoking and lung cancer.

Let us quote some further details for the light they shed on various
aspects of the cancer problem.

Breast cancer is uncommon in Japan, its mortality only a sixth of that
in England. Is this a built-in, i.e. genetic – immunity? When Japanese
emigrate to America, the incidence of breast cancer is still low in the second generation – suggestive of inbuilt rather than environmental factors.

Various factors have been considered. Prolonged breast-feeding is common in Japan, but if this acts as a safeguard against breast cancer it fails to account for the equally low incidence in unmarried Japanese women. Dietetic differences are another serious possibility. Japan has one of the lowest fat consumptions in the world, Western countries among the highest. Increased fat consumption by Japanese in America may well be relevant. Attractive as this proposition seems, it receives no support from the fact that in both world wars the low fat consumption of Central Europe did not lead to any decrease in breast cancer. Similarly cancers of colon, endometrium, ovary and prostate are all low risks in Japan, but take on the higher risk of the West after emigration to U.S.A.

Hormonal factors must also be considered. The breast, uterus, ovary and prostate are all subject to hormonal influence. Urinary hormone excretion has been investigated and the patterns in native Japanese women differ from those who have migrated to the U.S.A. Again a correlation with dietary fat seems plausible for we know that. oestrogenic hormone tends to be retained in adipose tissue. It is very interesting to find that myocardial infarction is also uncommon in Japan, but becomes commoner after emigration, once again suggestive of dietary factors.

Table 1.2 (p. 8) gives much food for thought. Half of all the cancers in British men are seen to originate in only two tissues, the surface linings of the respiratory and gastro-intestinal tracts. And about three-quarters in either sex arise at only five sites. Of these, the lung, bowel, skin and urinary tract are all subject to constant assaults from the environment with consequent repeated demands for repair, – i.e. chronic irritation in a broad sense (see p. 12). It is no surprise to find that these tissues are liable to develop multiple cancers.

The cervix is another site where environmental stress is crucial. Cancer of cervix is virtually unknown in celibate women (e.g. nuns) and much commoner in the married than in the single. There is some association with multiparity and we used to think cancer was due to trauma in childbirth and could be prevented by good obstetric care, but this is not so. A far more important relation lies in sexual intercourse, particularly promiscuity. Age at commencement of intercourse is important – if it is under 20 years. the risk is double compared with over 20 years. The number of partners is also relevant – remarriage after widowhood or divorce increases the risk, while the incidence in prostitutes is six times the normal. Circumcision of the male has long been thought to have some association with the freedom of Jewesses from cervical cancer. In India the incidence in communities which practise circumcision (Moslems) is less than in those which do not (Hindus). It seems to be a question of standards of personal hygiene. Circumcision is part of this, but not an essential part as shown by the Parsees – a religious sect in India – who are not circumcised but have high hygienic standards and a low rate of cervical cancer. Poor hygiene probably accounts for the increasing incidence found as we descend the social scale.

The conclusion seems to be that social factors are of prime importance in cancer of the cervix and it is estimated that improvement in hygiene (both male and female) could abolish perhaps four-fifths of the present incidence. But the evidence from different races is still doubtful and inconclusive. Circumcision in itself is now thought not to be protective. Even poor Jewesses rarely develop cervical cancer – so there may after all be some genetic factor at work. Certainly the evidence does not justify advising universal circumcision.

The association between lung cancer and smoking, particularly cigarettes, is now notorious. Cigars and pipes, although not free from risk, are much less dangerous. It is an unquestionable statistical fact that the risk of developing lung cancer increases in proportion to the amount smoked daily. Among men smoking 25 or more cigarettes a day, one in eight will die of lung cancer. At 35 cigarettes a day, the risk of cancer is 45 times as high as in non-smokers. Yet it is still on the increase, is now the commonest and most serious cancer in men, and becoming more frequent in women.

Atmospheric pollution is probably a contributory cause, and may help to explain the higher incidence in urban areas. This explanation appeals to smokers and the tobacco trade, but if it was true, road workers and policemen would have a significantly higher incidence of lung cancer. In fact they do not, and smoking habits are a far more likely reason for the discrepancy.

Industrial respiratory irritants are often carcinogenic – e.g. arsenic, asbestos, chrome, nickel, radioactive materials (see p. 13). Another striking illustration is the high incidence of lung cancer in Mexican women due to smoke-filled kitchens from flueless stoves, and similarly in South African Bantu women from braziers.

### Early detection and cancer screening

Next to prevention, early diagnosis – preferably before the stage of symptoms – gives the best chance of success. Too many patients do not report symptoms to their doctors as soon as they could. This is a problem in health education and is discussed below. Here we are concerned with pre-symptomatic diagnosis. Although we use the word 'early', we must remember that when a cancer becomes detectable, it is always 'late' in the sense that most of its natural life will already have passed and there may already be hidden distant metastases. 'Early' is therefore a relative concept, of clinical application. An early breast cancer that is only just palpable (or perhaps picked up on mammography and not yet palpable) is a very different problem from a late growth that has been allowed to fungate and invade the chest wall, even though the 'early' tumour may already have numerous microscopic secondaries lurking in liver, lung and bone, and the 'late' tumour may have none.

A simple test for malignancy would be enormously helpful – say, a serological test as for syphilis, or a biochemical blood estimation. There have in fact been many such claims advanced, but none, alas, has been confirmed.

*Pre-symptomatic diagnosis* clearly involves a positive search – getting at 'well' people who would not otherwise consult their doctors or feel the need to submit to any examination or test. Cancer screening programmes of this kind have been launched in many places in recent years and we are now accumulating some experience of their possibilities and value. They may cover whole communities or populations, or selected groups thought to be 'at risk', e.g. workers in a certain industry or factory.

Mass screening, to be worthwhile, must be acceptable to the population concerned. It must not be too troublesome for the individual nor too difficult to organise. It must be supported by educational campaigns and good follow-up with repeat examinations at appropriate intervals and references of all detected and suspected cases for further investigation and treatment. Questions of expense and economic use of available resources must of course be carefully weighed.

Apart from simple self-examination, the available methods include:
1. Periodic medical examination.
2. Cytological examination.
3. Radiological examination.
4. Highly specialised techniques – thermography, radioactive isotopes, biochemical and hormonal estimations and ultrasonics. These are mostly still experimental and not – or not yet – suitable for mass surveys.

*Periodic medical examination.* This has achieved a limited popularity, especially in U.S.A., applied either to selected groups such as business executives or offered commercially to those able to afford it. In addition to ordinary clinical examination, it includes a variety of laboratory investigations (blood and urine), chest film, possibly barium meal, sigmoidoscopy etc. It is unavoidably costly and therefore unsuited to large-scale surveys.

*Cytological methods* differ from histological – the latter relate to cells organised in tissues (Greek 'histos' = tissue), the former to cells isolated singly or in tiny clusters (Greek 'cytos' = receptacle or cell). Growing tumours shed – or 'exfoliate' – cells from their surface and these can be fixed and stained on a slide and examined microscopically. The expert can recognise abnormal features of cancer cells, e.g. nuclear irregularities.

This technique of exfoliative cytology was perfected by Papanicolaou in U.S.A. Its greatest merit is that it avoids the drawbacks of surgical biopsy.

a. *Uterine cervix* – early cancer or pre-cancer can be detected by cervical smear (see p. 35). This is the most common, the most important, the most valuable application of cytological diagnosis.

b. *Urinary tract,* especially bladder. After centrifugation, cells deposited from urine are examined for evidence of malignancy. This technique is useful for screening, e.g. workers in the dye and rubber industries who are at above-average risk. The method is more acceptable than routine cystoscopy, though less accurate.

c. *Lung.* Cells from sputum may be detected as malignant and may make bronchoscopy superfluous.

d. *Stomach.* Gastric washings may yield cancer cells.

e. *Prostate.* Cells in the secretion obtained from prostatic massage may be malignant.

*Radiological examination* is also of great value. Examples are:

a. *Chest films* – for detection of lung cancer in surveys comparable to mass miniature radiography.

b. *Barium meal* investigation. In Japan, which has an exceptionally high incidence of stomach cancer, mobile teams with radiographic equipment have developed a comparable technique for mass miniature radiography.

c. *Mammography* is a recent technique which is undoubtedly able to detect many breast cancers months and even years before they can be felt.

*Thermography* depends on the fact that cancers as well as other lesions (especially inflammatory) have a greater blood supply than their surroundings and consequently a raised temperature. A 'heat picture' can be taken, using the infra-red rays emitted from the body surface, and abnormal areas detected. Breast cancers may be picked up in this way. The technique is difficult and has not been widely adopted. It is much less accurate than mammography.

*Evaluation of screen programmes.* No nurse or doctor is likely to dispute that early diagnosis is a good thing. The widest possible mass surveys would therefore seem to be the merest common sense. But they are expensive and time-consuming. What then can be learned from experience so far? As usual we must consider different cancers separately.

*Lung.* In view of the appalling current rise in incidence and mortality, this is the most urgent problem of all. In Britain the recorded deaths have increased thus:

    1910–1000      1946–8000      1966–27 000

Numbers have actually doubled since 1954 and are still rising. They are now in the region of 30 000 annually, and in men lung cancer is responsible for 1 in 12 of all deaths. One heavy smoker in eight will die of it. It actually accounts for 40 per cent of all male cancer deaths.

There have been several mass surveys, by radiography and/or sputum cytology, but the results of pre-symptomatic treatment have been little better than that given after symptoms have appeared. Mass radiography is relatively cheap, but sputum cytology is very costly in expert man-hours. The bitter fact is that 80 per cent of all patients undergoing surgical resection die with secondaries which usually precede radiologically detectable disease. In theory, earlier diagnosis should increase the small proportion without metastasis, but in practice it does not seem to reduce the ultimate mortality.

The conclusion so far must be that, until there is a marked improvement in the results of treatment, the case for routine mass radiography or sputum cytology is weak, both on medical and economic grounds. Exception should be made for middle-aged people with persistent cough and for heavy smokers – if only as a gentle reminder! Much better dividends could be expected from preventive measures if only they could be widely applied.

*Cervix.* Here the picture is brighter. The cervical smear is well established in many places as a routine procedure. With a specially shaped wooden spatula a surface scraping is made round the external os and the material transferred to a slide (Fig. 3.1). Experience in several countries has confirmed that cervical cancers are detectable many years before the symptomatic stage and earlier treatment gives better survival figures.

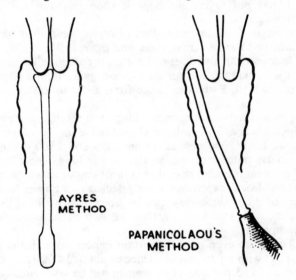

Fig. 3.1 Two methods of taking material for cervical cytology. *Left* – Ayre's spatula for scraping the surface of the external os. *Right* – Papanicolaou's method of aspirating fluid, with exfoliated cells, from vaginal fornix. (*Jeffcoate, Principles of Gynaecology, Butterworths*)

*Carcinoma-in-situ* (see p. 123-5) is of special interest and importance. It is found in 4 or 5 out of every 1000 apparently normal women over the age of 25. It is generally believed to be pre-cancerous, but not always. There is fairly good evidence that it may turn into true invasive cancer, but the proportion which do is uncertain and estimates vary from a quarter to two-thirds. Some workers question the whole relationship of carcinoma-in-situ to invasive cancer and consider that, even if some do become invasive, most never pass through a pre-invasive phase. In other words, the two lesions are quite distinct and not parts of a single process.

We must also appreciate that the discovery of early cervical (or any other) cancer by routine examination of 'well' people will still not completely prevent cancer deaths. For instance, in one series of early invasive cancers so discovered, almost 1 in 6 later died of cancer.

In spite of these doubts, there is now no question that mass screening can give results. In those centres where intensive screening programmes have been successfully maintained for years, the incidence of invasive cancer has fallen dramatically and advanced cancers are almost non-existent. Our most reliable evidence comes from British Columbia (Canada) where the incidence of clinical cancer of the cervix dropped by over a half in 11 years. But the acid test is, of course, the effect on mortality. Is the ultimate death rate from cancer any lower? So far in British Columbia it has not fallen; we hope it soon will and are anxiously awaiting later figures.

Our knowledge of the natural history of cervical cancer is still so poor that it is difficult to assess these facts and figures. We can at least say that early detection can and does mean a great reduction in suffering and benefit for the individual. But an elaborate organisation is required and the total cost is high. Estimates range from £300 to £1000 per cancer detected.

We must await further evidence and long-term results before we can be certain whether cervical cytology is justifiable on a national scale. Meanwhile we have 5000 new cases annually and 2500 deaths. Treatment is obviously much more successful than in lung cancer, but a mortality of 50 per cent is higher than that in most countries with comparable health services. Local experiments are justified and nurses have an important part to play, since they can be trained to perform the smears themselves, as well as taking part in the associated educational and publicity campaigns.

*Breast.* This is an even more important cancer numerically speaking (Table 1.2, p. 2) with an annual incidence of about 14 000 new cases and 10 000 deaths – i.e. 5 per cent of all women will be affected at some time of their lives. The mortality from breast cancer, unlike most other cancers, is not falling; there is actually a slight rise.

*Self-examination* for a lump in the breast is the simplest and most obvious means of early detection. Intensive public education has been achieved, especially in parts of U.S.A., but initial enthusiasm and regular self-examination soon fade. Though many tumours can be and have been discovered early in this way, the ultimate results in terms of mortality have been frankly disappointing. In general the larger the growth, the worse the prognosis. Yet in one series of really small breast cancers (about 1.5 cm, no bigger than a hazel nut) in which the results up to 10 years after operation were relatively good, more than half eventually died of their cancer. One-and-a-half centimetres is near the limit of ordinary clinical detection and we must therefore be very cautious in any claims we make.

*Mammography* has some definite advantages and should be very useful. It is of little value in the small fibrous breast, but very helpful especially in the large breast. It can reveal clinically impalpable cancers up to four years before they become clinically evident, including lesions less than a centimetre in diameter. It should be used as a supplement to clinical examination, not as a substitute, since the results of both combined are distinctly superior to either alone. An important large-scale survey is in progress in New York. Initial mass screening showed nearly three cancers in each 1000 women and at operation a lower incidence than usual of axillary node invasion. This was a very favourable feature which is certainly encouraging. On the other hand the false positive rate was high, since two-thirds of the suspected lesions submitted to biopsy proved non-malignant. It is too early to assess the long-term effect on mortality and the trial continues.

Looking at the possibilities on a national basis, we must bear in mind – quite apart from how many women could be persuaded to submit to it – the expense of X-ray equipment, radiographers, radiologists, doctors for clinical examination etc. There would be several negative biopsies for each cancer detected, and the cost would be about £1000 per cancer found. The resources for anything but small local experiments in Britain simply do not exist and are unlikely to exist for a long time yet. In a few years' time the New York survey should give us the answer to the key question – does early diagnosis improve survival? If it does, then large-scale surveys would be justifiable. Even in New York, however it has now been decided that the results do not justify continuing the programme on the same scale. Some useful lessons have been learned, but it is certainly not the answer to the breast cancer problem.

*Stomach.* In Japan mass miniature radiography has had some appreciable success and discovered early cancers which were successfully resected in two-thirds of cases, a remarkably high proportion. The method is justified in countries with an incidence of gastric cancer as high as that in Japan. In the West the incidence has declined markedly, perhaps due to improved diet.

*Large intestine and rectum.* Cancer of the large bowel is now the second commonest lethal cancer in Britain, exceeded only by lung cancer. Screening has been practised in some cancer detection centres in U.S.A., by clinical examination and sigmoidoscopy plus barium enema if indicated. Early cancers were discovered, but this type of examination is not likely to be acceptable on a large-scale – even if the resources were available which is not the case at present.

Reliance must still be placed on immediate investigation of suspicious bowel disturbances or episodes of rectal bleeding, especially in middle age and after.

## Prevention of cancer

Prevention is not the same thing as early detection, though the subjects overlap both with each other and with cancer education, so we may usefully consider them together.

At a recent cancer congress one authority asserted that 90 per cent of cancer could be prevented, at least in principle. We needed new organisation, application of new knowledge, a better liaison between public, research worker, and doctor. This is a large and optimistic assertion. Even if we do not know 'the cause' of cancer, we actually know more about the causative mechanisms of some types of cancer than of many other diseases which are more or less controllable, e.g. diabetes. Complete knowledge of causes is not essential for prevention or control. For instance, we know that protecting the skin from contact with pitch will prevent pitch warts and cancers, and that abolition of cigarettes would prevent most lung cancer, even though we do not know precisely how these irritants work.

The known causes include various physical and chemical factors and some of these we have already mentioned – ultra-violet and ionising radiations, soot, lubricating oils, dyes, asbestos. Occupational exposure is known to be responsible for some cancers of skin, lung, bladder etc. Medical inspectors of factories are well aware of the potential dangers and nurses employed in industrial work can play an important part in education and reassurance of workers, in medical examinations and protective measures (clothing, respirators etc.) and periodic checks (e.g. urine samples for detection of bladder cancer – see p. 33). The number of people involved is relatively small, but there is good reason to suspect that environmental carcinogens essentially similar in action play a large part in cancer production, especially in modern industrialised urban conditions, which include general atmospheric pollution.)

Occupational cancers form only a small proportion of human neoplasms, but their importance far exceeds their incidence. They are excellent models of chemical carcinogenesis and give us invaluable leads for prevention. New chemicals and industrial processes are pouring out, but their dangers are difficult to recognise because of the long latent interval before cancer production becomes apparent. It is only reasonable to assume that there are many unrecognised occupational hazards in our midst.

A host of other possible factors have been incriminated such as pesticides, fertilisers, creosote (which is carcinogenic for mice), though the evidence for many of these is slender. Dietetic factors are certainly important, either non-specific malnutrition and avitaminosis allowing absorption of environmental carcinogens (possibly responsible for the high incidence of liver cancer in Africa) or specific but unknown irritants. Suspicion has rested on cooking processes, overheating of fats, food additives (saccharin, cyclamates, preservatives, colouring and flavouring agents) and on smoked foods (the smoke contains the same type of carcinogen as tar and tobacco). Gastric cancer is rife in Iceland where consumption of smoked food is high. But for obscure reasons it has been declining in incidence for the past half century, both here and in U.S.A., while colon cancer has not changed. There is also some correlation between diet and hormonal patterns and changes in dietary fat intake may help to explain differences in breast cancer in Japanese women (see p. 30).

Hygienic factors have been illustrated in cancer of the cervix and penis (see p. 31). Improved oral and dental hygiene is probably responsible for the fall in cancer of the mouth. Septic and jagged teeth used to be associated with cancer of the tongue. Chronic alcoholism, now declining but far from extinct, is also accompanied by a high incidence of cancer of mouth, pharynx and oesophagus and in New York half the patients with oral and oesophageal cancer are alcoholics. The contraceptive pill has also been a subject of speculation. Whether it has any effect either way – by increasing or decreasing cancer incidence (e.g. in breast or cervix or ovary) still remains to be seen.

These lists could be extended, but we clearly have enough knowledge already to reduce the influence of at least many known carcinogens if only the knowledge was properly applied.

## Cancer education

There is a public 'image' of cancer as 'an incurable disease'. In fact the terms are commonly used interchangeably. The natural reaction to this is fear and 'escapism' – a refusal even to face the possibility – till forced by serious symptoms such as pain or heavy bleeding. This attitude is understandable since most families will have had experience of terminal cancer in relatives, friends or neighbours. Cancer's ugly reputation is bound to persist – after all, it is only about a century since medical science stood helpless before the problem, and even now the overall results of treatment are not brilliant.

It is difficult for the layman to appreciate what can now be done – that something like a third of all cancers can be either 'cured' in the popular sense or controlled well enough to give patients an expectation of life not far from normal, and that good palliation of symptoms can be achieved in most cases.

At this point it may be noted that even nurses are liable to undue pessimism. For in the nature of things we require their services to care for the failures of treatment rather than the successes. Successful treatment is apt to go unsung, while failure cries out loud.

So great is the fear of cancer that doctors tend not to give the full details to patients to avoid causing them excessive worry. One result of this is that many patients successfully treated are unaware of the real nature of their trouble and cannot spread the good news. Only the failures are left to spread bad news. It is not generally realised that there are many thousands of cured cancer patients leading normal lives. And it is difficult to appreciate the difference between radical and palliative treatment, so that the inevitable eventual failure after palliative therapy is interpreted as a failure of attempted cure. This subject is difficult and controversial, but must be an everyday concern to nurses in contact with these patients. It is impossible to lay down general rules. Cases will vary in maturity, personality, family background, economic circumstances etc. and each patient is a separate problem.

This fear of cancer is a potent factor in causing delay in diagnosis. If I have cancer – an incurable disease – I prefer not to know it or not to have it confirmed, so I won't go to a doctor. It may not be put consciously in these terms of course, but this sums up the psychological mechanism. For example, medico-social surveys have shown:

1. Most women are well aware that a lump in the breast might be cancer.

2. Most patients, after detecting such a lump, delay many weeks or months (and even years) before seeking advice.

3. Patients who knew the possible significance actually delayed longer than those who did not.

4. The most important factor in delay was the belief that cancer is inevitably fatal.

Cancer is seen as a threat to one's personal integrity in the most literal sense. It is our task to get the public to regard cancer as one serious disease among others, to be feared no more, yet no less. Nurses have an important part to play in this campaign of enlightenment, whether inside or outside hospital. But we must realise that we are dealing with something that has deep roots in the human psyche. We are all subject to the illusion of immortality. And the evidence shows that even doctors do not usually get earlier treatment than their patients. This is presumably true for nurses also. Clearly it is not just a matter of simple ignorance; it is much more deep-seated. So let us temper science and rationalism with charity and realism, and appreciate that public education will not accomplish miracles. And we must make no extravagant claims which would only discredit our activities and make a bad situation worse.

There has been a good deal of educational activity, notably by the American Cancer Society, in an effort to enlighten the general public and encourage people to undergo routine checks (e.g. cervical smears, chest X-ray) and report leading symptoms at an early stage. Radio, television and films have been used as well as books, pamphlets and discussion groups (Women's Institutes etc.). Of all these media, the small group is best where individuals are not inhibited from asking questions freely, and can even discuss their fears and phobias. Nurses are often called on to play their part in these activities and should be well briefed with background knowledge, both of cancer and human nature. It is uphill work and its results are not easy to assess, but it is possible to lower the barriers of ignorance and prejudice among whole communities in this way. Some of the myths surrounding cancer can thus be dispelled, but cancerphobia is only one of the many and widely prevalent neuroses of our time, and even if we succeed in removing this particular worry from an individual he may merely switch to a cardiac neurosis instead.

Apart from pre-symptomatic checks, educational drives seek to induce people to come to their doctor with early symptoms or signs. It is customary to stress the significance of the following:

1. Unusual vaginal bleeding or discharge, especially intermenstrual or post-menopausal (cancer of uterus).

2. A lump or thickening in the breast – or neck, armpit, groin or elsewhere (breast cancer, Hodgkin's disease etc.).

3. A sore or ulcer that does not soon heal – on skin, lip, tongue etc. (epithelioma).

4. Unusual indigestion or difficulty in swallowing (cancer of stomach or oesophagus).

5. Blood in the urine or from the rectum (cancer of bladder or bowel).

6. Spitting or vomiting blood (cancer of lung or stomach).

7. Unusual cough or hoarseness (cancer of lung or larynx).

8. A change in regular bowel or bladder habits (cancer of colon, bladder, prostate).

9. Bleeding or a change in size or colour in a wart or mole (epithelioma, malignant melanoma).

It is most important to emphasise that *not one of these is at all diagnostic of cancer*. Blood from the rectum is commonly due to 'piles', a lump in the breast may be a simple cyst, vaginal bleeding may come from a benign polyp (or even an old forgotten pessary!). But any of them might be the first indication of cancer and should be investigated. Unfortunately early diagnosis does not guarantee cure, and it is foolish and misleading to make such a claim. We have already noted that a cancer is often present for years before even pre-symptomatic detection is possible. In any particular case of apparently early cancer we can rarely be sure whether metastasis has already occurred but in a significant proportion of cases earlier diagnosis can mean the difference between life and death. This alone would justify our efforts. We can further claim that late diagnosis will worsen the chances of either cure or useful palliation, and will carry a high risk of increased suffering.

The object of public education is to change the climate of opinion, to dispel the belief that cancer is necessarily fatal and replace it by the knowledge that cancer is often curable or at least manageable. An informed public opinion is our best ally against cancer and it is worth stressing such points as the excellent chances in clinically early cancers of skin, larynx, cervix, rectum, tongue etc., and the prolongation of life and comfort (and even working capacity) in other cases where complete control cannot be achieved. Even if the cancer mortality figures are to be marginally improved – and this is the most we can expect in our present state of knowledge – the benefits of early diagnosis and treatment are still real and significant in many cases and of considerable value to the patients and families concerned.

'Cancer education' alone is not an ideal for psychological reasons. Ideally it should be incorporated in a wider programme of health education, beginning at school and including the elements of personal and public hygiene, with the stress on preventive measures and healthy living, fresh air, proper diet, exercise and improvements in our social environment. At the moment the biggest impact of all would result from an effective campaign to reduce smoking, especially cigarettes, but here the psychological problems are notorious. It is worth mentioning that the incidence of lung cancer in doctors is now falling – from 1954 to 1964 it fell by 30 per cent, while in the general population it rose by 25 per cent. Doctors are about the only section of the community where consumption of cigarettes is known to have decreased. Is the same true of nurses, one wonders, especially as cigarette smoking by women generally is increasing. In fact the rate of increase of lung cancer in females is now higher than that for males.

We quoted above an estimate that 90 per cent of cancer is preventable. At the moment we should certainly be able to prevent about 40 per cent of cancer deaths in men (mainly lung) and 10 per cent in women (mainly cervix). Even though we are still ignorant of the intimate mechanism of cancer and of the way the body normally controls cellular proliferation, and though each type of cancer has still to be considered separately and empirically, there is good reason to believe that a considerable proportion of the remaining cancers should be ultimately preventable and that major advances will probably be made by the end of this century. Medical science can pin-point many causative factors and estimate the risks, but implementing an effective policy of prevention calls for governmental action and social and personal discipline. This means that public education on a broad front is essential and progress will be slow. It may be regrettable, but most people are reluctant to take good advice about health if it interferes with their pleasure, otherwise there would be far fewer sweets eaten and far fewer cigarettes smoked! (There may be some food for thought in the fact that among the religious sect of Seventh Day Adventists in U.S.A. – who prohibit tobacco and alcohol and consume little meat, fish, tea or coffee – there is a low incidence of cancers of lung, mouth, larynx, oesophagus and cervix.)

Note. The health risk from lung cancer to our affluent cigarette-smoking society in the 20th century is comparable in scale to the ravages of tuberculosis in the slums of the industrial revolution in the 19th century. It is a melancholy fact that the revenue from tobacco is enough to finance a third of the National Health Service. It is legitimate to wonder why the government does not apply differential taxes to discourage cigarettes in favour of less dangerous cigars and pipes (as is done in Holland) or does so very little to control the brain-washing of susceptible youth by tobacco advertisements.

A recent writer has estimated that over 5000 hospital beds in this country are occupied by victims of cigarettes – chronic bronchitis, lung and other cancers, and cardiovascular disorders – i.e. 4.5 per cent of all hospital beds. In other words, in an 800-bed hospital, a ward of 36 would be filled by the results of cigarette smoking, and the cost to the Health Service of this proportion of beds totals £60 million annually.

In U.S.A. it has been estimated that almost 20 per cent of working days lost between the ages of 17 and 64 may be ascribed to cigarettes.

# 4. Physical Principles and Equipment

*In Nature's infinite book of secrecy*
*A little I can read.*

Shakespeare (Antony and Cleopatra)

To understand what goes on in a radiotherapy department, it is desirable to have a nodding acquaintance with a few aspects of modern physics. This is not difficult and needs no mathematics. The medical radiotherapist has to qualify in radiological physics and works with professional physicists for treatment planning, dosage estimation, calibration of equipment etc. For the nurse's purpose such detail is not necessary, but a little knowledge will add enlightenment and interest. Some of the details may appear complicated at first, but will be useful for reference.

Radiotherapy means treatment by ionising rays (radiations) – ionisation is explained on p. 47. These rays are of two kinds:

1.Waves        2. Particles

*1. Waves.* Most of these rays – X-rays, gamma rays – can also be called waves, and we can picture them in wave form, Fig. 4.1. The distance from crest to crest – or trough to trough – is the wave-length and this can be measured. There is a wide band – or spectrum – of rays in nature, of varying wave-lengths, ranging from a fraction of a millionth of a millimetre (short-wave radiation) up to many thousands of metres (long-wave radiation) – Fig. 4.2.

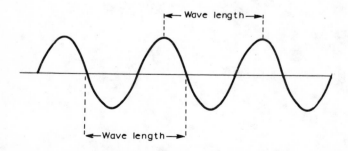

Fig. 4.1 Waves and wave-length.

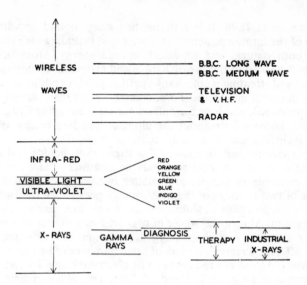

Fig. 4.2 The electromagnetic spectrum of waves and wave-lengths.

It is the difference in wave-length that gives the rays their particular and characteristic properties. In the middle of the range lie the wave-lengths of ordinary visible light (a mixture of all the colours of the rainbow) to which our retina is sensitive. All the other rays are invisible to us. Just beyond the red (long-wave) end of the visible spectrum lie the infra-red rays (ordinary heat rays, from gas or electric fires etc.), and just beyond the violet (short-wave) end lie the ultra-violet rays (from sunshine, mercury vapour lamps etc.)..

In radiotherapy we use the very much shorter wave-lengths of the X-ray and gamma ray regions. Note, we shall not be concerned with the medical use of ultra-violet, infra-red, short-wave diathermy – nor with ultra-sound. These treatments are usually done in the physiotherapy, not the radiotherapy, department. In radiotherapy the radiations used are all of the ionising type (see p. 47); the others mentioned are of much longer wave-length and not ionising.

2. *Particles* include:

(a) alpha particles (rays); (b) beta particles (rays); (c) electrons; (d) neutrons; (e) protons.

These are described below. They are all ionising.

### The structure of matter

Our knowledge of X-rays, gamma rays and the various particles is recent, beginning with Roentgen's discoveries in 1895 and the Curies' isola-

Note – alpha, beta, gamma ($\alpha$ $\beta$ $\gamma$) are the first three letters of the Greek alphabet.

tion of radium in 1898. It is a fascinating story, bound up with the un-ravelling of the intimte structure of matter and including radioactive sub-stances (both natural and artificial), atomic energy, atom bombs etc. Medically it has led to the use of X-rays and radioactive materials for the diagnosis and treatment of many pathological conditions, of which cancer is the most important. To understand what these agents are, how they are produced, and how they affect matter – including living matter – we need to know a little about the ultimate 'building bricks' of all sub-stances, including our own body cells.

*Chemical elements and the atom.* All matter-solids, liquids and gases – is composed of basic chemical materials or *elements*. There are about 90 different elements in nature, and matter is usually composed of com-binations of two or more of them. About 99 per cent of the earth's crust consists of oxygen, silicon, aluminium, iron, calcium, magnesium, sodium and potassium. Almost the whole of organic living matter is composed of only four elements – carbon, oxygen, hydrogen and nitrogen.

Each different element consists of huge numbers of tiny identical units called *atoms*. Atoms are too small to be observed singly by visual means. The diameter of an atom is about $10^{-8}$ cm. This is a convenient way of writing 1/100 000 000 cm – i.e., one hundred million atoms side by side would occupy a length of one centimeter.

*The electrical nature of matter.* Atoms used to be regarded as hard in-divisible spheres of which about 90 different kinds existed. Within the last 60 years we have learned that atoms are composed of a few simple par-ticles combined in different ways. The unravelling of the structure of the atom has gone along with the development of our knowledge of the nature and properties of the radiations with which we are concerned here.

We now know that not only is matter fundamentally electrical in its nature, but also that electricity itself is atomic in structure. In the 18th century two kinds of electrification were recognised, and it was supposed that two electrical fluids existed – positive and negative – which were equal in quantity in an unelectrified body and so neutralised each other. We now recognise fundamental units of positive and negative electrical charge.

Figure 4.3 shows how we now picture atoms. The simplest kind is that of ordinary hydrogen, found in all living tissues. Its structure resembles the earth with its moon – a relatively large and heavy centre with a tiny particle circling it all the time. The centre part of an atom is called the *nucleus*. Its size varies from one kind of atom to another, but is always very small compared with the whole atom. The diameter of the nucleus is only about one ten-thousandth of the atomic diameter. Most of the volume of an atom is therefore 'empty space'.

The atom is an electrical structure. In the case of hydrogen, the nucleus consists of a single particle carrying a single positive charge, marked by a positive sign (+). It's 'moon' is also a single and very much tinier particle, carrying a single negative electrical charge, marked by a negative sign (–). This negative particle is called an *electron*. Electrons are the fundamental units of electricity, and an electric current is essentially a stream of electrons.

Every atom consists of a small positively charged nucleus around which negatively charged electrons move. Surrounding the nucleus is a system of electrons, each moving round in some definite orbit or shell. The total number of such electrons is equal to the number of positive charges carried by the nucleus, so that the whole atom is electrically neutral. We can compare the structure of an atom with the solar system. It is like the sun surrounded by moving planets. Actually the ratio of the sun's diameter to the orbit of the most distant planet is about the same as the ratio of the atomic nucleus to the whole atom.

The nucleus of the hydrogen atom with its single positive electrical charge is called a *proton,* balanced of course by the single negative charge of the circling electron. The next simplest atom is Helium (Fig. 4.3), whose nucleus contains two protons and is correspondingly balanced by two orbital electrons. The helium nucleus also contains two additional particles called *neutrons,* so called because they carry no electrical charge and are therefore electrically neutral. As we continue up the scale of chemical elements, the general plan remains the same, but the nuclei contain increasing numbers of protons and neutrons and correspondingly increased numbers of electrons circulating in multiple shells. For example, the neon atom in Fig. 4.3 is seen to contain 10 nuclear protons, 10 nuclear neutrons, and 10 outer electrons in two shells.

*Ionisation.* The electrons whirling round the outside of an atom are rather loosely attached and can be knocked off. The atom then loses a unit of negative electrical charge and is left with an unbalanced surplus of positive charge. The dislodged electron is usually caught on a neighbouring atom, which thus acquires an unbalanced extra unit of negative charge. These abnormal fragments – one electrically positive due to the removal of electrons, the other electrically negative through the addition of extra ones – are called *ions,* and the process is called *ionisation.*

Ion is Greek for 'moving thing' – for these charged particles are easily movable under the influence of an electric field.

All the radiations dealt with in this book are ionising radiations, because they knock electrons off atoms in their path, e.g. in living cells. This ionisation causes physical and chemical changes in cells, and these changes are responsible for the resultant biological effects (see p. 64).

*Isotopes.* The really fundamental and characteristic difference between the different chemical elements lies in the electrical charge on the nucleus – i.e. the number of protons which is always the same as the number of orbital electrons. If the charges on the central nuclei of two atoms differ – i.e. if they have different numbers of protons – then the number of electrons in the outer regions of the atoms differs, and also the arrangement of these electrons. It is this arrangement which determines the chemical

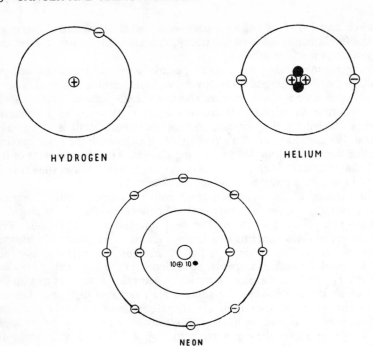

Fig. 4.3 Diagrams of atomic structure.
$\oplus$ = Proton, $\ominus$ = Electron, $\bullet$ = Neutron.

nature and behaviour of the atoms.

Each element always has the same number of protons in the nuclei of its atoms, but may have different numbers of neutrons. Ordinary hydrogen, for example (Fig. 4.3), has only one proton in its nucleus, but there are other hydrogen atoms with one proton and one neutron – 'heavy' hydrogen or deuterium – and still other hydrogen atoms with one proton and two neutrons – tritium. These three varieties of atom are all hydrogen and behave as such chemically, since they all have the same orbital electron structure – i.e. only one electron. And the same holds for the varieties of all other chemical elements which have the same number of orbital electrons.

These varieties of a particular element with different numbers of nuclear neutrons are called *isotopes* of that element. Greek 'iso' means 'equal' and 'tope' means 'place', i.e. they occupy the same place in the chemical table of elements.

The total number of particles in the nucleus – protons plus neutrons – is thus characteristic of each isotope and is conveniently used to designate it. The isotope of hydrogen with one proton and two neutrons is referred to as Hydrogen-3 or abbreviated as H-3 or $^3$H. Other common examples of interest to us are:

Cobalt-60 or $^{60}$Co; Iodine-131 or $^{131}$I; Phosphorus-32 or $^{32}$P.

### Radioactive isotopes (or Radio-Isotopes)

Most isotopes in nature are stable — i.e. they remain permanently unchanged. Some elements, however, especially very heavy ones — heavier than lead — with large nuclei and many more neutrons than protons, are unstable — i.e. their nuclei undergo a process of spontaneous re-adjustment or transformation, with partial disintegration so that they change into isotopes of other elements.

In this process they emit ionising radiation, and this emission of radiation accompanying nuclear transformations is called *radioactivity*.

Naturally-occurring radioactivity is found mostly in a few heavy elements, e.g. radium. However we can now produce artificial radioactive isotopes of all the chemical elements by subjecting them to bombardment by neutrons in the nuclear reactor, a sort of 'atomic furnace' where atomic energy is produced (as well as material for atom bombs).

These radiations, whether from natural or artificial radio-isotopes, are of three kinds, named after the first three letters of the Greek alphabet: 1. Alpha rays (or particles). 2. Beta rays (or particles). 3. Gamma rays.

*1. Alpha rays.* These are particles composed of two protons and two neutrons packed tightly together. A glance at Fig. 4.3 shows that this is the same as the nucleus of a helium atom. Alpha particles are, in fact, bare helium nuclei.

They are the least penetrating of the three — their range in air is about 10 cm — and easily absorbed, e.g. by a very thin layer of paper. They cannot penetrate the skin, but are intensely ionising over the short distances they travel and so can be very damaging to tissues if the substance which emits them is absorbed in the body (see p. 13-14).

They are not now used in radiotherapy but must obviously be considered in questions of protection.

*2. Beta rays.* These are streams of fast-moving particles which are actually electrons. Their penetrating power varies considerably according to the particular isotope emitting them but it is much greater than that of alpha rays. They can easily penetrate thin metal foils and in soft tissues can travel distances ranging from small fractions of a millimetre up to about one centimetre, producing ionisations in their path.

Beta-emitting isotopes may be used for beta-ray therapy (p. 61). If we wish to confine the betas so that they do not emerge from the container of the isotope emitting them — as we do in most kinds of radium treatment — this can be simply done by screening with thin layers of metal (p. 54).

*3. Gamma rays.* These are exactly the same as the more penetrating of the X-rays (Fig. 4.2). The difference is merely in name — when they come from radioactive substances we call them gamma rays, but when they are produced by electrical machines we call them X-rays.

They differ fundamentally from alpha and beta radiations, as they are not particles but waves of the same type as light and radio waves (Fig. 4.2) but with different properties because of their very much shorter wave-length.

Their penetrating powers are very much greater than those of alpha or beta rays. They can reach the deepest tissues in the body, even penetrate the whole thickness of the body – hence their great value in treatment.

Serious protection problems obviously arise when we deal with gamma-emitting isotopes (Ch. 7).

### Radioactive decay; half life

Radioactive substances like radium are always losing matter and energy because of the radiations they give out – i.e. they are constantly destroying themselves or *decaying*.

If an atomic nucleus loses some of its substance in this way, it is easy to see that a new species of atom might be formed – i.e. a different chemical element (the old alchemist's dream of changing base metal to gold!). This is particularly true of the heavy naturally-occurring radioactive isotopes. *Radium* is a good example; it undergoes a whole series of transformations, as the daughter isotopes are themselves also unstable and give rise to further radioactive isotopes (Fig. 4.4). The first such isotope produced by radium is the gas *radon* (p. 54) and the whole series of transformations in the course of time ends up with the production of ordinary stable lead.

To measure the rate of decay and to compare one radio-isotope with another, we use the *half-life*, i.e. the time taken by the material to decay to half its original activity, Fig. 4.5. In this period of time, half the number of atoms in any particular sample will have disintegrated. *The half-life is a constant and characteristic value for each and every radioactive isotope.*

If we call the original amount 100 per cent and if the half-life is, say, a week, then after one week there will be 50 per cent of its radioactivity left. At the end of the second week half of this 50 per cent will have disappeared, leaving 25 per cent, and after the third week half of the 25 per cent will have gone, leaving $12\frac{1}{2}$ per cent ... and so on.

The rate of decay is very variable. For radium it is about 1600 years, so that for practical purposes we can regard its activity as virtually constant over any person's lifetime. Others decay faster, e.g. radiocobalt (much used for gamma ray therapy) takes over five years to decay to half strength. Radioactive iodine (also in regular clinical use) takes eight days. *Unit of measurement of radioactivity.* This is the *Curie* – abbreviated as Ci – after Marie Curie, the famous discoverer of radium. One curie signifies the breakdown of 37 000 million atoms per second of any particular radioactive substance in question. This is not an arbitrary figure,

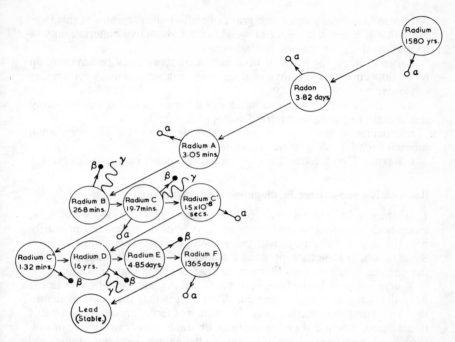

Fig. 4.4 Radium and its disintegration products, with the radiations emitted at each disintegration. The figure inside each circle is the half-life.

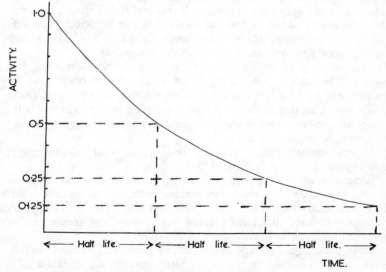

Fig. 4.5 Radioactive decay and the meaning of 'half-life'.

but arose historically since one gram of radium disintegrates at this rate. Note that it is not a measure of weight of a radioactive material, only of its radioactivity or rate of breakdown.

Large sources, for instance in cobalt beam units, may be anything up to 10 000 curies. It is convenient to have smaller sub-units for smaller amounts:

millicurie = mCi = one thousandth of a curie – a useful unit for many therapeutic techniques requiring isotopes.

microcurie = $\mu$ Ci = one millionth of a curie – for the very small amounts used in diagnostic tracer tests.

( $\mu$ is the Greek letter 'm' – pronounced 'mew', rhymes with 'new'.)

## Radioactive substances in diagnosis and treatment

*1. Diagnosis.* In medical work, radioisotopes – like X rays – are of great value both in diagnosis and therapy. This book is concerned primarily with therapy, but the diagnostic use of isotopes is now expanding rapidly. Since nurses in radiotherapy units are bound to meet many examples and the subject overlaps radiotherapy, a brief account may be useful.

*Tracer studies.* As we have seen above, all the isotopes of any element have the same chemical behaviour. This means that they can enter into the same chemical reactions and the same metabolic processes and paths in the body, whether they are unstable or stable – i.e. radioactive or not. Biological processes therefore cannot distinguish between stable and radioactive isotopes of the same element. The fate of a substance of biological interest can therefore be followed or traced if we can label it by introducing a radioactive tag in place of its normal stable atomic isotope.

The radiations emitted by the radioactive tag can be detected outside the body by highly sensitive instruments capable of detecting and measuring very tiny quantities of radiation (see below).

The patient will of course receive some small radiation dose, but because of the extreme sensitivity of detection, the isotopes used for tracer tests can be given in such small quantities that the radiation effects are negligible. Valuable clinical information can be obtained in this way.

Tracer studies are now the most frequent application of radioisotopes in medicine. A few examples:

a. Thyroid studies. This is the commonest tracer study, for investigation of thyroid function (see pp. 191-3).

b. Bone scanning. Radio-strontium or technetium is taken up in bone, and in increased quantities in various pathological conditions, including secondary deposits from malignant growths. These may therefore be detected at an early stage, even before the appearance of radiological changes in a diagnostic X-ray film.

c. Brain scanning. Primary or secondary tumours and other abnormalities can be detected in the brain after intravenous injection of a suitable isotope.

d. Liver scanning can be carried out in a similar way and show up secondary deposits.

2. *Therapy*. Radioactive substances are used for therapy in two different forms, which are referred to as 'sources' − i.e. sources of ionising radiations:

    i. Sealed sources − permanently and completely enclosed in metal containers.

    ii. Unsealed sources − in liquid form in solution.

i. *Sealed sources*
    a. Large sealed sources. These are the gamma ray beam units. The most important are:

        Cobalt beam unit    Caesium beam unit

    b. Small sealed sources. Applicators for localised gamma ray treatment to limited regions of tissue:

Radium  
Cobalt } needles and tubes  
Caesium  
Gold grains  
Iridium − Wire and pins

Beta-ray applicators for superficial treatment of limited areas, in thin-walled containers which allow betas to emerge:

Strontium applicators  
Yttrium − rods or pellets.

ii. *Unsealed sources*. Almost entirely for beta radiation. Some emit gamma rays also, but this fraction of the total radiation is of minor importance.

Iodine } Systemic use − intravenous or oral. Distributed  
Phosphorus throughout body by normal metabolic processes.

Gold } Intracavitary instillation for maligant effusions in  
Yttrium serous cavities.

*Note* − all the radioactive isotopes used as diagnostic tracers are also unsealed sources.

### Detection and measurement of radioactivity

To control the use of unsealed sources we need to detect and measure their radioactivity, e.g. in samples of blood or urine, or the content of an organ in the body, or in material spread around in accidental contamination on hands, clothing etc.

The commonest detection and measuring systems are:

1. *Geiger counter*. This measures electronically the ionisation produced by the radiation in a gas.

2. *Scintillation counter*. This counts the flashes of light produced by radiation in crystals.

The most important instrument is the *Scintiscanner* used for organ scanning – so called from the to-and-fro motion in the recording process. The picture it produces shows the presence and distribution of the isotope and is called a scintiscan (see Fig. 11.2, p. 198). Its use is well illustrated in the technique of radio-iodine investigation in thyroid disease.

3. *Gamma camera*. This is a more advanced form of apparatus giving more rapid visualisation of whole organs or parts of the body, and the picture produced is called a scintigraph or scintigram.

*Small sealed gamma ray sources*

The commonest type is a needle or tube containing radium (or one of its substitutes), Fig. 4.6.

Radium needles are thin hollow metal containers with sharp pointed ends to pierce tissues; the other end carries an eyelet for threading with silk. One or more thin-walled cells, filled with radium in powder form, occupy the central cavity. The metal wall is commonly a platinum alloy with iridium for increased mechanical strength; it has to absorb the beta rays emitted by the radium and allow only the gammas to emerge. If the betas were allowed to emerge, they would do destructive damage to the tissue immediately adjacent to the needle in a very short time, long before the time needed for the penetrating gammas to do their work, and local necrosis would result. Since the needle must be as thin as conveniently possible, a very dense metal must be used to give the maximum of filtration for its thickness. Platinum fulfils this requirement (so does gold). It has other advantages too – a very high melting point, so that it is not destroyed if accidentally thrown into the incinerator along with dressings from the ward; and since it is non-corrosive it can easily be cleaned.

Radium needles are made in various convenient lengths – between 2.5 and 6.0 cm with diameters just under 2 mm. They contain 1, 2 or 3 mg of radium. Special forceps and pushers are needed for their insertion (Fig. 8.16, p. 140).

Radium tubes are essentially similar to needles, but shorter, of larger diameter and need no pointed ends as they are not for direct insertion in tissues. Their radium content is usually higher – 5 or 25 mg or more.

*Gold grains or radon seeds – an alternative to radium*

Radon is a daughter product generated by the natural decay of radium (Fig. 4.4). It is a gas, unlike the solid form of radium, but emits the same radiations as radium. The other special difference from radium is its short half-life – 3.8 days – as opposed to the 1600 years of its parent radium.

In previous years it was widely used in thin tubing, in the form of 'radon seeds' of short length, but these have now been almost entirely

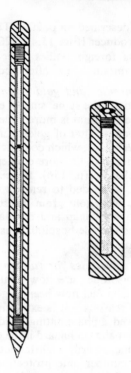

Fig. 4.6 Showing the construction of radium needles and tubes. Needle, cell filled (*left*). Tube (*right*). (*Paterson, X-ray and Radium Treatment of Malignant Diseases, Edw. Arnold*)

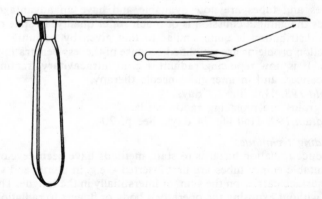

Fig. 4.7 Radon seed introducer or '*gun*' (*Paterson, X-ray and Radium Treatment of Malignant Diseases, Edw. Arnold*)

replaced by *gold grains* (described on p. 202). They may be inserted into tissues with a special introducer (Fig. 11.4 p. 202) and left permanently buried, forming harmless foreign bodies after their radioactivity has decayed to a negligible amount – i.e. after about a fortnight.

### Comparison of radium needles and gold grains

The treatment is essentially the same, since it employs the same type of gamma rays in each case. Radium is more widely useful as its radiation intensity is virtually constant. That of gold decreases steadily, falling to half its original value in 2.7 days, which complicates dosage calculations. Grains, on the other hand, may be more convenient for some awkward situations such as the bladder (p. 156). If needles were used there, a second operation would be needed to remove them.

Patients can go home with gold grain insertions or surface moulds, since they are comparatively cheap and not dangerous if lost, whereas radium cannot be allowed outside hospital. This saves hospital beds and possibly patients' working time.

### Radioactive isotopes as substitutes for radium

Several artificial radioisotopes are now available which can replace natural radium, which has in fact now been largely discarded. Ra–226 is objectionable for several reasons – it is expensive; it emits a radioactive gas (radon) with long-lived alpha-emitting solid daughter products and consequent ingestion or inhalation hazard if the container is fractured; its gamma ray energy is unnecessarily high for localised radiotherapy and so needs expensive and cumbersome protection.

1. *Cobalt-60* Half-life 5.3 years.

Needles and tubes, as well as other shapes such as spheres and rings can easily be produced. Cobalt 'beads', can be packed e.g. into the uterine cavity, like Heyman radium tubes (see Fig. 8.15, p. 137).

2. *Caesium-137*. Half-life 30 years.

Needles and tubes are now available and have an advantage over radium as the gamma emission is of much softer quality. In spite of this, the dose distribution is quite similar to that given by radium.

Protection problems are simplified because of the less penetrating gamma rays. It is now replacing radium, e.g. in intracavitary treatment of uterine cancer, and in interstitial needle therapy.

3. *Gold-198*. Half-life 2.7 days.

Gold grains are replacing radon seeds.

4. *Iridium-192*. Half-life 74 days. See p. 204.

### Afterloading techniques

To reduce radiation hazards to staff, methods have been developed in which suitable empty tubes are first inserted – e.g. in uterus and vagina, or on a surface carrier on the skin, or interstitially in the tongue. This can be done without exposing the operator's body or fingers to radiation. The position of the tubes can be checked by radiography and corrected if necessary. The radioactive sources are then inserted within the pre-arranged tubes by remote control, once again with minimal radiation exposure of working personnel.

This afterloading technique is under trial, e.g. for cancer of the cervix, Fig. 4.8. The sources are several hundred times more active than in the ordinary technique (p. 128) and the treatment is given daily for a short period in a specially protected room.

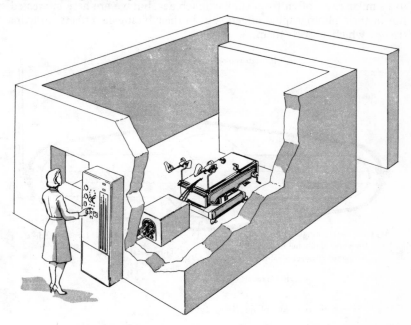

Fig. 4.8 After-loading technique. The patient is in a radiation-protected room. Radium sources are inserted, by remote control from outside the room, into tubes previously positioned in the patient. At the end of each treatment the sources are withdrawn into the safe. (The Cathetron, *courtesy T.E.M. Instruments Ltd.*)

## X-Rays

X-rays were discovered by the German physicist Roentgen in 1895 and are often called Roentgen rays. Although they occur naturally, e.g. in outer space – on earth they are mostly produced by electrical machines. Otherwise they are of exactly the same nature as gamma rays. *Production.* Figure 4.9 shows the manner of X-ray production. A heating current is passed through a filament and at a high temperature electrons are 'boiled off'. The high voltage across the tube then speeds these electrons so that they hit a metal target with an impact of such violence that rays are produced from the disturbed atoms – mostly heat, but a proportion of short wave-lengths too, including X-rays.

In megavoltage units, more sophisticated methods of accelerating the electrons are used to increase the violence of their impact and so produce shorter wave-lengths, but the fundamental principle is the same.

X-rays are used in diagnostic radiology because they can penetrate matter to a variable extent, and the rays emerging from the other side of the body then affect a photographic film which can be developed – like a snapshot – to show 'shadow pictures', e.g. of bones. In radiotherapy we use similar rays, often from similar machines, but we are here interested, not in their photographic effects, but in their biological effects on living tissues which absorb them.

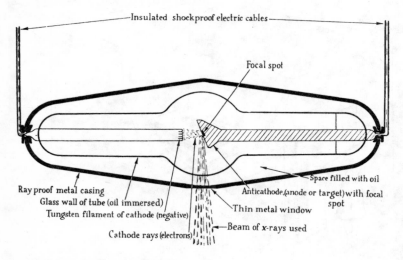

Fig. 4.9 Schematic diagram of an X-ray tube.

## Equipment

Some of the X-ray units in a radiotherapy department are quite similar to those in the diagnostic X-ray department, but the more powerful units now used are very different. They differ in the penetrating power of the X-rays – i.e. their ability to reach not only surface tissues but also tissues deeper in the body. The penetrating power depends on the electrical pressure in the machine, and this is measured in volts. X-ray units vary in their voltage.

To form a mental picture, we can compare electrical pressure with the water pressure of a waterfall – the higher the waterfall, the greater the pressure. A low-voltage machine will produce rays of comparatively long wave-length (Fig. 4.1, p. 44) which may be absorbed almost entirely by the skin, while high-voltage rays, i.e. of short wave-length – may penetrate so deeply that some emerge from the opposite side of the body.

According to their penetrating power, which in turn depends on wave-length, beams of rays are described as varying in *quality*. We speak of them as relatively *soft* or *hard*. The harder they are (i.e. the shorter the wave-length) the more penetrating the ray.

The ordinary voltage in the electric mains in this country is about 240. In a typical diagnostic X-ray machine it is about 80 000 volts – abbreviated as 80 kV (k for kilo, Greek for 'thousand'). For therapy we use X-rays generated at widely different voltages according to the different degrees of penetration required:

1. Superficial therapy – from 10 to 140 kV.
2. Deep therapy – about 250 kV. Sometimes called 'orthovoltage'.
3. Supervoltage or Megavoltage therapy – over one million volts.

Mega – Greek for 'great' – is used to denote 'million(s)'.

*Note* – the gamma rays of cobalt beam units are also in the megavoltage range.

## Superficial therapy units

These are used mainly for skin lesions, both malignant and non-malignant.

*Grenz rays*. Grenz is German for 'boundary', and these rays are so called because they lie on the border between the hardest ultra-violet rays and X-rays (Fig. 4.2, p. 45). They are in the 10-15 kV region, very soft easily absorbed, and therefore fairly safe, as they cannot damage subcutaneous structures. One widely used unit is the 'Dermopan' set made by the firm of Siemens, which works at voltages adjustable between 10 and 50 kV. Other so-called Contact sets work at 45-60 kV.

The most generally useful kind of superficial X-ray unit is one working between 60 and 140 kV. This can treat skin lesions, e.g. epitheliomas, too thick to be safely treated by Grenz or Contact units. An example is the KX10 (or GX10) unit, which can cope with almost the whole of the superficial therapy in any department.

## Deep therapy units

Until about 10-15 years ago these were the standard machines doing the great bulk of the work. At about 250 kV, the beams of X-rays they produced gave reasonably deep penetration (Fig. 4.15) so that lesions deep in the body could be treated. Most of our experience in radiotherapy has been acquired on this basis, and most departments still use a unit of this type. They are now on the way out, since there is little or nothing they can do that cannot be better done by the new megavoltage and gamma ray beam units with their superior powers of penetration and other advantages (see below).

## Megavoltage units

There are several types, working on different principles, but the most important is now the linear accelerator (Fig. 4.10). The energy of the X-ray beam is measured, not in thousands of volts, but in millions and their penetration is correspondingly greater (Fig. 4.15). Units are now available in the 4-20 million volt region.

Another but less common type of unit is called the *Betatron,* and can produce X-rays at 15-20 MV or more.

Megavoltage units, especially linear accelerators and/or cobalt beams, are coming increasingly into use and are handling nearly all except superficial treatments.

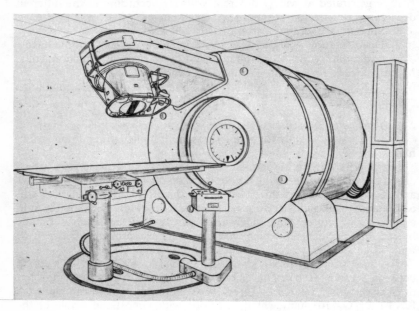

Fig. 4.10 Linear accelerator for megavoltage therapy. (*Courtesy of Radiation Dynamics Ltd.*)

## Gamma ray beam units

A gamma ray beam unit (Fig. 4.11) consists essentially of a thick-walled heavy metal container with an aperture through which the gamma ray beam emerges. Techniques for using the beams are the same as for X-ray megavoltage beams.

An alternative name is *telecurie therapy.* (Greek 'tele' = 'far' or 'distant', as in telephone) so called because the radioactive source is at a comparatively long distance from the patient.

Not many radioactive isotopes are suitable for this purpose. Formerly radium itself was used, but this is scarce and costly. It has now been superseded by radiocobalt or Co-60. Its half-life is reasonably long, 5.3 years, so that the source in the unit does not need to be renewed too frequently as it decays – in practice every two or three years. The gamma rays are equivalent to megavoltage X-rays at about two million volts.

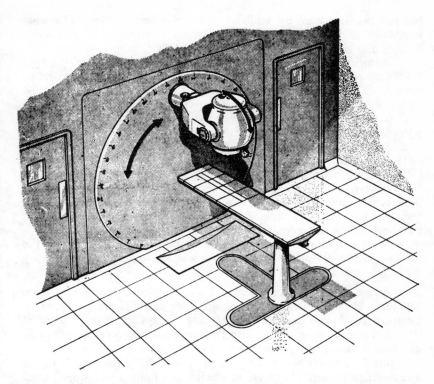

Fig. 4.11 Gamma ray beam unit (radioactive cobalt) for megavoltage therapy. (*Courtesy T. E. M. Engineering Ltd.*)

Radiocobalt units are widely used now, and this is actually the most important application of radioisotopes in cancer therapy.

Another radioisotope used in gamma ray beam units is caesium-137, though to a much lesser extent. This has a half-life of about 30 years, and the gamma rays are equivalent to X-rays at about one million volts – i.e. intermediate between deep X-ray and cobalt beam therapy.

### Particle therapy

Various ionising particles may be used in therapy:
1. Beta particles (rays).
2. Electrons.
3. Neutrons.
4. Protons – so rare that we shall not deal with this use.
1. *Beta rays*. These can be used in several ways:
   a. *Surface therapy,* in surface applicators (often called plaques). Radium was once used in this way for skin lesions (e.g. rodent ulcers),

but has been replaced by artificial radioactive beta-emitters. The most important of these is Strontium-90, which is particularly useful for treating the surface of the eye (see pp. 203-4).

b. *Intracavitary therapy*. This is a form of 'internal surface' therapy. Radioisotopes in solution can be injected into serous cavities, pleural or peritoneal. Malignant deposits on pleural or peritoneal surfaces can thus be locally irradiated and this can often control serous effusions.

Gold ($^{198}$Au), phosphorus ($^{32}$P) and yttrium ($^{90}$Y) can be used for this purpose but have now largely given way to intracavitary cytotoxic drugs.

c. *Systemic therapy*. Common examples are the use of radio-iodine ($^{131}$I) in hyperthyroidism and thyroid cancer, and radio-phosphorus ($^{32}$P) in polycythaemia (see Ch. 11).

d. *Interstitial therapy*. This is an uncommon use. A beta-emitter can be directly injected into tissues (in solution) to give intense, very localised radiation to a small volume. Radio-gold has been used in this way to treat, e.g. inoperable prostatic cancer.

Another and more frequent example is the use of yttrium-90, in the form of small solid pellets or rods, or in a paste, to destroy the pituitary gland (see pp. 203, 210).

2. *Electron therapy*. Electrons are physically identical with beta rays. The term 'electron therapy' is used when the particles are produced by electrical machines. Instead of producing X-rays by striking a target (Fig. 4.9) the electrons emerge directly from the tube, and electron beams can then be used like X-ray beams for therapy.

Figure 4.12 shows how the dosage in tissue differs from deep X-ray or megavoltage beams. The range of electrons is limited and stops rather abruptly. For example, at 15 million volts the dose is fairly uniform from the surface down to a depth of 4 cm (90 to 100 per cent) and then falls very rapidly, reaching 50 per cent in another 2 cm. A dose distribution limited in depth in this way can be very useful in some conditions, e.g. to treat with a single field tumours just below the surface, while sparing the deeper tissues to a large extent – compare Fig. 4.15.

Electron therapy has been much used in some centres, but not widely in Britain. It is doubtful whether it has any real advantages over other types of treatment.

3. *Neutron therapy*. Neutron beams suitable for therapy have recently become available, and developmental and experimental work is in progress. Clinical trials have begun, but it is too early to assess the value of this form of treatment.

There are certain technical radiobiological advantages which lead us to believe that neutron therapy may be particularly useful in resistant cancers where there is oxygen deficiency (see p. 82).

## Measurements and dosages

The biological effects which interest us here are brought about by physico-chemical changes in living cells, and these result ultimately from the ionisations produced by the rays when they are absorbed. From the physical aspect, therefore, the use of X-rays and all the other types of ionising radiations involves merely the production of a certain amount of ionisation under suitable conditions in a particular region of the body.

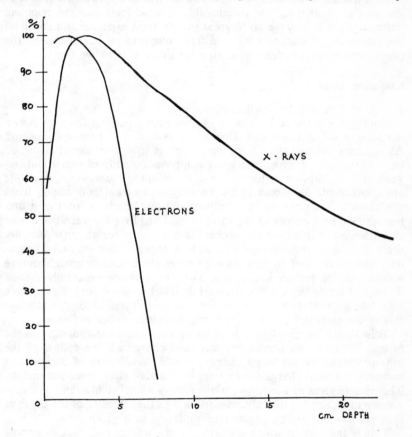

Fig. 4.12 Comparison of depth-dose curves for electrons and X-rays at 15 million volts.

But how much ionisation? – and what are suitable conditions? To put treatment on a scientific basis, we must be able to measure amounts of ionisation, and for measurement we need a unit – just as for radioactivity. Radiation measurement is an exact science – in fact, far more exact than in any drug or other therapy. When we administer a drug we know the total quantity given, but we seldom know much about its relative distribution in the patient's various organs. In radiotherapy the amount and distribution of dosage (i.e. ionisation) is crucial to the success or failure of our treatment and we can now determine this with great accuracy in almost all cases.

We need to know these details of dose and distribution because we want to damage cancerous tissue without inflicting excessive damage on normal tissues. Otherwise we would run the risk of destroying a cancer at the cost of destroying the patient also – or at least causing crippling damage. That is why we go to great trouble (and expense) and enroll all the resources of science with help from our invaluable colleagues, the physicists, to secure this knowledge for every patient we treat.

## Radiation units

*1. The Roentgen* (also spelled Röntgen)

Consider a beam of X-rays or gamma rays emerging from an X-ray machine or cobalt beam unit. How much radiation is there in the beam? As it passes through the air, it meets – and is to a small extent absorbed by – the atoms of which the air is composed, mainly nitrogen and oxygen. The absorption is due to ionisation of these atoms – i.e. electrons are knocked off the outer regions. This involves a transfer of energy from the beam to the air – rather like warming our hands in front of a fire, transferring heat energy in the form of infra-red rays from the fire to our skin (though in this case the process is not one of ionisation). Actually these dislodged electrons move off at high speed – they are called secondary electrons – and in turn dislodge other electrons from neighbouring atoms, causing further ionisations. The electrons are eventually slowed down and are finally caught and held on nearby atoms, forming negative ions. The general effect can be pictured as a short trail of ionisations, and this is the essential process occurring in matter under radiation.

This ionisation gives us a method of measuring the radiation in the beam. The ions produced carry electrical charges. If we collect all the ions produced by the beam in, say, a cubic centimetre of air, we can measure the total charge they carry, by suitable electronic instruments. This charge gives us a measure of the energy absorbed in each cubic centimetre of air, and is directly proportional to the intensity of the beam at that point – i.e. to the quantity of radiation in a given time.

This is the way in which we arrive at the unit of radiation dose now adopted. It is called after the discoverer of X-rays, the Roentgen – abbreviated to R. The same unit applies to gamma rays, which are of the same nature, but not to radiations of a different nature, the particles (alpha, beta etc.).

The Roentgen accurately measures the radiation in a beam of rays as they emerge from their generating source. It is clearly very important that engineers and physicists should be able to measure the output of these machines. The output measured over a certain period of time gives us the amount of radiation to which a patient is exposed. This is the *exposure* and is measured in roentgens.

## 2. The rad

What we want to know for therapy is the amount of radiation absorbed, not by the air through which the beam passes, but by the body tissues.

The unit of *absorbed dose* is the Rad.

It measures the amount of energy imparted to matter by ionising radiation. It is therefore a more fundamental unit for our chief purpose, the dosage to tissues. Moreover the roentgen can only be applied to X-ray and gamma ray beams, whereas the rad can be used for all types of ionising radiations.

If the atoms of the absorbing material differ from those of air, their energy absorption from the beam of rays will also differ. Now the atoms of soft tissue in the body (e.g. muscle) are very similar to those of air, so that the exposure (in roentgens) will measure fairly accurately the absorbed dose (in rads). But in the case of hard tissue – especially bone – composed of different atoms, the energy absorbed may be significantly greater depending on the voltage of the radiation, while in fat the energy absorption may actually be less.

## 3. The rem

This is another unit which has special importance in matters of protection. It takes into account not only the absorbed dose in rads, but also the fact that some radiations are more effective than others in producing biological effects. For example, the heavily ionising particles, neutrons and alpha rays, have much greater effects, rad for rad, than X-rays or beta rays.

To take account of this, a dose in rads must be modified by appropriate numerical factors, so as to arrive at a figure representing the biological effect of the dose delivered. This gives us the '*dose equivalent*'. *Note* – for practical purposes, in as far as they concern the subjects in this book, the rad, the roentgen and the rem can be taken as equal in magnitude and therefore interchangeable.

## Dose distribution in tissues from X-ray and gamma ray beams

A radiotherapist who is to use a beam of rays must have full information about the distribution of dose which the beam will produce in the body under the actual conditions of treatment. This information lies in the province of the hospital physicist, an essential member of a radiotherapy department.

*Applicators.* The beam must be restricted to the area defined for treatment, usually the skin. In superficial and deep therapy, this is achieved by an applicator. This is a cylindrical or cone-shaped attachment to the X-ray tube, Fig. 4.13.

In megavoltage therapy, applicators are not normally used because in most cases it is important not to have anything touching the patient (see below). The field is defined by adjustable diaphragms near to the source of the beam – as in Fig. 4.13 but without an added applicator.

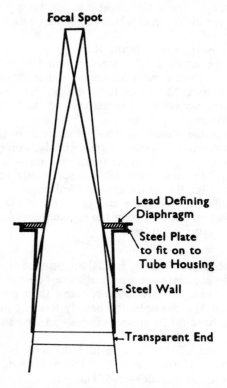

**Focal Spot**

**Lead Defining Diaphragm**

**Steel Plate to fit on to Tube Housing**

**Steel Wall**

**Transparent End**

Fig. 4.13 Diagram of X-ray treatment applicator, showing attachment to X-ray tube. The beam of X-rays is emitted from the Focal Spot – compare Fig. 4.9. (*Paterson, Treatment of Malignant Disease, Edw. Arnold*)

### Depth dose and isodose curves

By means of direct measurements in a suitable medium – a substitute for human tissue is called a 'phantom', e.g. a water-tank – the physicist can plot the distribution of dose produced by a beam of any particular quality, area and shape. The dose is examined from the surface downwards, both at the centre and edges of each field, and charted as percentages of the highest dose, which will be at or near the centre of the surface.

The highest dosage is labelled 100 per cent and all the other doses are expressed as percentages of this – i.e. percentage depth dose.

The result is a set of curves (Figs 4.14, 4.15) drawn through points of equal dosage. These are called *isodose curves* – Greek 'iso' means 'equal' – and are basic tools for treatment planning. They will clearly vary with the quality of radiation concerned. There is a vast difference between superficial therapy at 45 kV (Fig. 4.14) and supervoltage (Fig. 4.15). The depth dose at 2 cm in the former is 5 per cent compared with over 90 per cent in the latter.

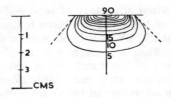

Fig. 4.14 Isodose curves at 45 kV.

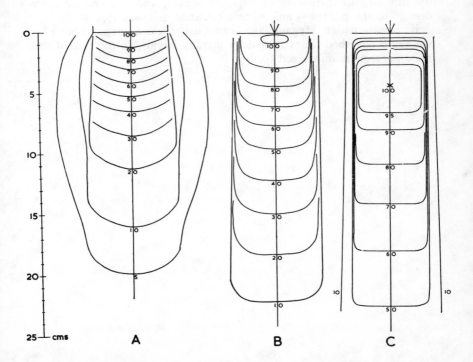

Fig. 4.15 Comparison of isodose curves from (A) 200 kV, (B) 2 MV, (C) 20 MV.

*Advantages of megavoltage*

a. *Depth dose*. The obvious superiority of megavoltage lies in its greatly increased depth dosage.

b. *Build-up*. A glance at the figures shows that, in contrast to superficial and deep therapy, the maximum dose is received, not at the skin surface but a little below it — just how far below depends on the voltage. This is because the secondary electrons move mainly in a forward direction so that the ionisation 'builds up' to a peak below the surface.

This is a very important advantage of supervoltage in therapy for it means that the effect on the skin for a given tumour dose is much less than in deep therapy at 250 kV. It is important for the patient since skin reactions with megavoltage are much less troublesome and interfere much less with schemes of treatment (see p. 88). And it is one main reason why we do not use applicators with closed ends, as in deep therapy; if we did, the advantage of the skin-sparing build-up would be lost.

c. *Beam definition*. It can be seen that megavoltage beams have sharper, better defined edges. This means more exact concentration on the tumour, better sparing of adjacent organs, and less general body dosage to the patient — and so less radiation sickness (pp. 96-7).

d. *Bone damage*. Megavoltage beams cause less damage to bone for the same absorbed doses than deep therapy beams, so the risk of late bone necrosis is minimised (p. 96).

# 5. Principles of Treatment and Dosage

*Stimulate the phagocytes.*
George Bernard Shaw (The Doctor's Dilemma)

## General assessment and choice of treatment

Once a diagnosis of malignancy has been reached, some crucial decisions must be made:
1. To treat or not to treat.
2. To give radical or palliative treatment.
3. Which line of treatment to use – surgery, radiation, hormones, cytotoxic drugs – or a combination of these.

Very exceptionally, the decision may be to give no treatment – beyond sedatives and ordinary nursing care, e.g. if the growth is hopelessly advanced, or the type of cancer is known to be unresponsive. In such cases it is psychologically better not to attempt specific treatment.

*Assessment before treatment*
In every case we need to gather all relevant information about the patient in general and the growth in particular:
   a. General condition – age, coincident disease etc.
   b. Extent – how localised is it? how much invasion has occurred? are there lymph-node or distant metastases? This information is conveniently summarised where possible by clinical staging.
*General condition.* It is important to assess the patient's fitness for any drastic procedure. Old age, coincident diabetes, cardiac failure, hypertension, obesity etc. may rule out a hysterectomy for cancer of body of uterus, or radical radiation for bladder cancer.
*Extent.* Local, regional or distant spread is assessed by:
   1. Clinical examination – especially for accessible cancers, such as skin, mouth, cervix, breast. This includes palpation of regional lymph--node areas to detect enlargement, e.g. in the neck for mouth and throat cases, in axilla and above the clavicle for breast cases etc.
   2. Radiography – X-ray films of chest for secondaries in lungs, skeletal survey for secondaries in bone, intravenous pyelography (I.V.P.) for investigation of kidneys and ureters, lymphography for lymph-node involvement in pelvic and paraortic areas.
   3. Instrumental endoscopy – bronchoscopy for lung, cystoscopy for bladder, sigmoidoscopy for colon etc.

4. Isotope scans – radioactive tracer studies may detect primary or secondary growth in bone, brain, liver etc. (see pp. 52-3).

*Type.* Histological examination may be needed for diagnosis in a doubtful case. If there is no clinical doubt, e.g. in many basal cell carcinomas of skin – biopsy is often omitted. Sometimes biopsy before treatment is not practicable and histology must wait for the surgical specimen, e.g. after nephrectomy.

Histological grading may provide valuable information about the degree of differentiation of a growth and its liability to metastasis; its possible importance in choice of treatment has been mentioned (p. 28).

When the relevant investigations in these lines have been completed, we have to consider whether treatment is to be radical or palliative.

### Radical and palliative treatment

a. *Radical treatment* means the attempt to remove all the malignancy present. Staging of a growth is a logical approach in deciding whether treatment should be radical. In general, only stages 1 and 2 are suitable for radical surgery. Early stages are also the most suitable for radical radiation, but later stages are not ruled out, e.g. a Stage 3 cancer of cervix, with malignancy confined to the pelvis, is unsuitable for radical surgery but often suitable for radical radiation.

With very few exceptions, radical treatment means either primary surgery or primary radiation – or both – with radiation given either before or after surgery. Occasionally cytotoxic drugs may be included as part of radical treatment, but if so they will usually be a subsidiary part.

For surgery the growth must of course be operable – it must be considered possible to remove the whole of the primary mass with a safe margin. In some sites it is also possible to remove in the same block of tissue the lymphatic vessels and regional lymph-nodes. This will include any early lymphatic metastases, e.g. in radical mastectomy, the breast is removed with underlying muscle and the axillary lymphatic contents; in radical (Wertheim's) hysterectomy, the uterus and appendages are removed with as much as possible of the pelvic lymphatic tissue.

Radical radiotherapy similarly attempts to destroy the whole of the primary growth and may include the regional nodes.

b. *Palliative treatment* is used if radical treatment is considered impracticable because of age, debility or extent of spread – especially if there are known to be distant metastases. In general, these cases will be in Stage 3 or 4. The aims of palliative treatment are:

1. To relieve symptoms, e.g. pain, bleeding, cough – arising from primary or secondary growth.

2. To forestall or heal ulceration or fungation or pathological fracture of bone.

3. In general – to improve the quality of the rest of the patient's life.

In radical treatment heroic measures are justified, even if the strain on the patient is severe, as it often will be, for the stakes are life and death.

But in palliative treatment we are trying, not primarily to prolong life, but to make it more bearable and we are not justified to impose any severe strain. Treatment should be reasonably short, radiation reactions minimal. There should be no general upset.

Any of the four agents can be used for palliation. *Surgery* may be required for:

a. Obstruction, e.g. transurethral resection in prostatic cancer, colostomy in bowel cancer.

b. Pain, e.g. nerve block, section of posterior roots or sensory tract in the spinal cord, amputation of a painful bone sarcoma on a limb.

c. Paraplegia – laminectomy for relief of pressure on the spinal cord by a tumour mass.

d. Fixation of a pathological fracture by pinning.

e. Local removal of a fungating mass, as a toilet procedure, e.g. residual breast cancer.

*Radiation* is even more widely useful for palliation. Here are a few examples – others will be described in later chapters:

a. Relief of symptoms in lung cancer – haemoptysis, cough, pain.

b. Control of haematuria in bladder cancer.

c. Bone secondaries – relief of pain and local healing.

d. Cerebral secondaries – improvement in neurological symptoms.

e. Improvement or healing of ulceration or fungation in cancer of skin, breast etc.

*Hormones* and *cytotoxic drugs* are now used extensively for palliation in advanced cases. These are described in Chapters 12 and 13.

*Surgery or radiotherapy?*

The choice between these may be easy or difficult. The following factors will influence the decision:

1. Site        3. Radiosensitivity
2. Operability    4. Histology
           5. Clinical experience

These factors overlap, and some have already been discussed above.

1. *Site*. Some lesions are definitely unsuited to primary radiotherapy, e.g. all the gastro-intestinal tract from stomach to rectum; operable growths of breast, ovary, kidney, thyroid, lung; intracranial gliomas, meningiomas (see pp. 83-4).

2. *Operability*. Some lesions are clearly inoperable, e.g. breast cancer with deep invasion of chest wall.

3. *Radiosensitivity* (see p. 87 and Table 5.1, p. 81).

a. Low sensitivity of the growth. As a rule some lesions are so unresponsive to radiation that surgery is the only real hope of cure – e.g. osteosarcoma, fibrosarcoma.

b. High sensitivity of normal tissue. This may be the limiting factor – e.g. if it were not for the great sensitivity of normal intestinal epithelium, some bowel cancers would be treatable by radiation.

4. *Histology*. The degree of differentiation is relevant. Very undifferentiated (anaplastic) growths are more liable to invade and metastasise than well-differentiated growths. This factor should weigh in the balance, though not necessarily be decisive in itself. For example, if biopsy of a Stage 2 cancer of cervix shows high anaplasia, surgery is unlikely to be curative and radiation would be preferable.

5. *Clinical experience*. This is really the most important criterion of all and it incorporates all the above factors. Knowledge accumulates on the basis of recorded and sifted experience. Hence the great importance of cancer registration, follow-up of patients, and accurate recording of results – including side-effects, complications and survival.

For example an early mass of Hodgkin's disease or lymphosarcoma is easily removable by surgery, but new regional or distant lesions are virtually inevitable sooner or later, so that even enthusiastic surgeons rarely advocate this. In contrast, the results of radiation for malignant melanoma are usually so poor that surgery should always be the method of choice if possible.

All this is not to say that the choice between surgery and radiotherapy is always clearcut – far from it. Other factors may be involved. For example, in rodent ulcers of the face (the commonest site) the cosmetic results of radiation may be poor (they are always rather unpredictable) and this may determine the choice of surgery, especially in women.

In some cases, good results can be obtained by either method, e.g. in early (Stage 1) cancer of the cervix. Similarly with early cancer of the vocal cord of the larynx, excellent results follow both surgery and radiation, but radiation is usually preferred as it leaves the patient with a better voice.

In general, treatment policy varies between different countries and different individuals. There is no one method which is invariably 'best' and different methods give equally good results. Local resources and experience will often determine the choice. If radiotherapy is not readily available – it may be hundreds of miles away – surgery or cytotoxic drugs may be preferred. Individual doctors may have special experience in certain techniques and come to advocate them – not without justification, since any technique will give poor results in incompetent hands. For example, the criteria of operability in lung cancer may vary considerably and some thoracic surgeons will operate on border-line cases where others would not. Some chest clinics refer a large proportion of lung cancers for radiotherapy, others only a small percentage. It is the person that counts, not the scalpel or the machine.

Ideally patients should be seen at joint clinics where all relevant specialities are represented – surgeon or radiotherapist and (where indicated) gynaecologist, urologist, haematologist, dermatologist etc. In this way the best treatment can be jointly decided for the individual patient and clinical trials can be conducted. The ultimate test is the actual result. This is easy to say, not so easy to evaluate. Survival figures are the most obvious criterion of success, but not the only one, as we have already discussed.

## Principles of radiation treatment

### General medical principles

The radiotherapist is a physician first, a technical specialist second. If he is dealing with a small 'rodent ulcer' on the cheek of an otherwise healthy patient, radiotherapy is a comparatively simple matter − a few brief out-patient attendances suffice and though mistakes and complications can occur, ordinary care and routine thoroughness should ensure a smooth passage and complete success. Most patients however are not in this happy position, and though some may be able to receive treatment as out-patients others will need hospital care. Those treated by radioactive sources (radium etc.) will almost always have to be in-patients, if only for reasons of radiation protection.

The patient's general condition must always be considered first. He may need fluid replacement by intravenous drip, blood transfusion after haemorrhage, antibiotics for infection, concentrated nourishment and vitamins for malnutrition, diuretics for oedema, drugs for pain, spasm, cough etc. etc.

He may present a a medical or surgical emergency − cardiac failure, laryngeal obstruction, intestinal obstruction, compression paraplegia, pathological fracture etc. − and require the attention of the E.N.T., orthopaedic or neurological surgeon. However desperate and important these situations are, no new principles are involved and nurses will be familiar with their management. We shall deal only with those aspects which concern radiotherapeutic management which nurses will not meet· in other departments.

A course of radiotherapy, especially for radical treatment, is usually a strenuous affair for any patient, comparable to the strain of a major surgical operation. One or more of the various radiation effects described in the next chapter are bound to afford at least some discomfort and they may last for many weeks and sometimes even months before healing. The patient will need all the physical and moral support we can give him − not to mention his family also.

## Principles of radium treatment

Small sealed gamma ray sources have already been described (pp. 53-4) and this section applies both to radium and its substitutes − cobalt, caesium etc.

They are used in three principal ways:

       1. Intracavitary     2. Interstitial     3. Surface

*1. Intracavitary tubes* (less commonly needles) are inserted in natural body cavities. By far the most important clinical application is utero--

vaginal insertion for carcinoma of the uterus, especially cervix (pp. 128-132).

2. *Interstitial needles* surgically inserted and buried in the tissues, around and within malignant growth. Roughly one milligram of radium is needed for every cubic centimetre of tissue to be treated, and is left in for about a week.

This method is useful for small growths of easy access, where there is room for accurate manipulation, e.g. in the mouth, especially the tongue. It has the advantage of confining the radiation fairly strictly to the diseased area, so that only a minimum of normal tissue is irradiated. Hence a large dose can be safely given (see p. 139).

3. *Surface tubes* or needles are mounted on some form of applicator or mould which fits the treated part accurately — almost always the skin or mouth including lip. An example is given on p. 160.

This method is now outdated at many centres and has been replaced by X-rays.

Historically radium was used very extensively in the early days of radiotherapy — i.e. in the first half of this century — but has largely given way to X-rays after development of superficial and megavoltage machines and gamma ray beam units. The changeover goes on as equipment and techniques improve and different centres vary in their methods. Some still use surface radium for cancers of the skin, lip, hard palate etc., while others have completely abandoned this technique and rely on X-rays (or gamma ray beams).

Interstitial implants are also on the retreat. Once they were much used for floor of mouth, cheeks, fauces, bladder, breast, anus etc. but now they are confined to the small tongue lesion, with occasional use in vulva and breast so that very few implants may be done at some centres.

Intracavitary treatment was once used on sites such as maxillary antrum, nasal cavity and naso-pharynx, but is rarely used now except in the uterus and vagina where it still retains its pre-eminent role. Even here it is commonly supplemented by external radiation. Some workers foresee its eventual disappearance even for treatment of cancer of the cervix.

Substitution of X-rays for radium greatly lessens the problem of protection. Radium treatment always involves some degree of exposure for technical, nursing and medical staff, while X-ray therapy almost entirely avoids this hazard.

## Treatment planning for external radiation

For superficial and easily accessible lesions, such as a small epithelioma on the skin where the radiation field can be accurately positioned by eye, no special planning is necessary. The standard isodose distribution curves (Fig. 4.14, p 67) give us all the information we need Maximal dose is at the surface where we want it and falls off rapidly beneath the tumour so that deeper tissues are largely spared.

Contrast this with treatment of a deep-seated growth, e.g. a cancer of the oesophagus in the middle of the thorax, one of the deepest sites in the body. Clearly, a single field as in Fig. 5.1a – even megavoltage – will be inadequate. The highest dose would fall at, or just below, the skin surface, gradually diminishing at greater depths until at the oesophagus it would be perhaps a third of the maximum (Fig. 4.15, p. 67). To give a tumour lethal (cancericidal) dose with this single field would involve enormous doses to the chest wall, lung etc. and lead to early necrosis (p. 89). So we apply the principles of *multiple fields* and *cross firing*.

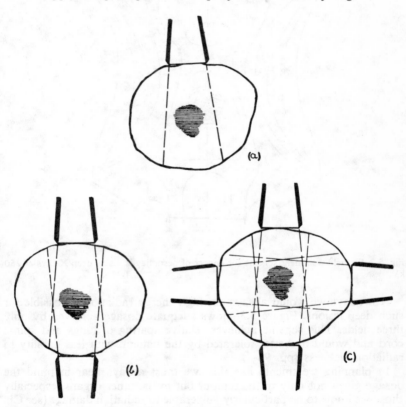

Fig. 5.1 X-ray fields and techniques: (a) single field; (b) a parallel pair; (c) two pairs of opposed fields.

A parallel pair of fields (Fig. 5.1b) would give too high a dose to the spinal cord, while four fields as in Fig. 5.1c would give too much to the lungs.

Figure 5.2 shows a six-field treatment scheme, using deep therapy at 250 kV. All six beams aim at the lesion, building up the dose at that point. It is seen to be 130 per cent as compared with 100 per cent at the skin surface – a practicable distribution, though still giving undesirably high dosage to the spinal cord.

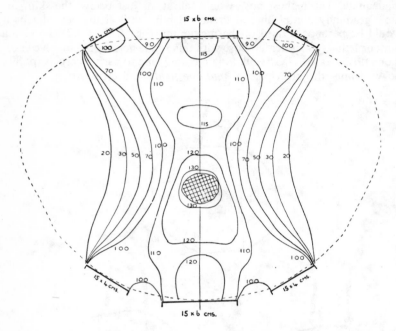

Fig. 5.2 Six-field treatment scheme for cancer of oesophagus, using deep X-rays at 250 kV.

Nowadays we would always use high energy radiation if possible for such deep lesions. Figure 5.3 shows adequate dosage achieved by only three fields. This scheme achieves relative sparing of lungs and spinal cord and would be better tolerated by the patient, with less liability to radiation sickness (pp. 96-7).

In planning treatments like this, we must always bear in mind the dosage given not only to the tumour but to the other organs, especially those we know to be particularly vulnerable to radiation damage (see Ch. 6). In this example we pay particular attention to the spinal cord and avoid using a directly posterior field passing straight through the vertebrae.

*Wedge filters.* Figure 5.4 – taken from a case of laryngeal cancer – shows a popular arrangement called a wedge pair. The adjacent edges of the beams are partly 'blacked out' by wedge-shaped filters. This gives a homogeneous dosage to a corner site, with maximal sparing of normal tissues.

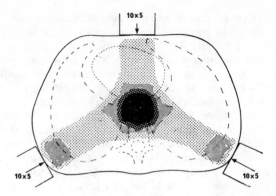

Fig. 5.3 Three-field megavoltage technique for cancer of oesophagus, at 4 MeV. Isodose symbols as in Fig. 5.4.

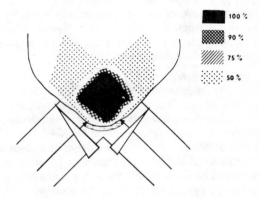

Fig. 5.4 A 'wedge pair' of fields.

### Tumour localisation and beam direction

The fields in Fig. 5.3 are narrow – only 5 cm wide – i.e. large enough to cover the growth with a small safety margin. It is a small field technique, designed to limit the volume of irradiated tissue as much as possible, consistent with inclusion of the whole cancer.

The smaller the volume irradiated, the higher the radiation dose we can safely give, and therefore the greater is the likelihood of achieving a cancericidal effect. Thus if the size of the treatment field is deliberately limited, the more important it will become to aim the beam accurately. This will be fairly simple on the anterior field, but more difficult on the two posterior oblique fields. Moreover, accurate direction of the beams must be ensured at every treatment session which may be daily for several weeks.

To achieve this, we must provide for:

a. Localisation of the growth in relation to the surface of the body or to some envelope or mould worn during treatment.

b. Beam direction by some mechanical or other arrangement.

*Localisation* is usually by radiography. In this case we would use a barium swallow. Another example is the bladder which can be visualised and localised after injection of a radio-opaque contrast medium. In other cases we might use natural bony points, e.g. the pituitary fossa – or insert radio-opaque foreign bodies, such as old radon seeds in the fauces etc.

In many cases, some form of 'shell' surrounding the body or part at the requisite level is the means of fixing the relationship of the growth to the surface and organising the direction of the beams in treatment. These shells are made of plastic material in the mould room of the radiotherapy department. This is a specialised business and it is usually necessary to make an accurate plaster cast of the part first, e.g. head and neck – and then mould the shell accurately on to this.

Nurses should pay a visit to the mould room and follow the process of construction of a cast and shell to fit the contours of an individual patient – a separate one must, of course, be specially made for each patient. The patient wears the shell at each treatment session and with its aid the therapy radiographer is able to use the special devices for ensuring the correct placing and angulation of the beam.

### Planning of dose distribution

To obtain the isodose plots of Figs. 5.2, 5.3, 5.4 we must first draw a life-size outline of the patient's body contour on paper and insert details of tumour position and other landmarks of importance, e.g. spinal cord and lungs. We then use isodose curves (Fig. 4.15, p. 67) and try various arrangements of fields, summating the doses as shown until we are satisfied we have obtained the best arrangement possible under the individual circumstances. This is a time-consuming business, but of vital importance and must be done for every single case where radical treatment is applied, for no two patients are identical in contour, dimensions etc.

This dose-planning is carried out in the clinical physics department and the nurse should see at least one case being planned in detail. After seeing the work done in mould room and physics department, nurses will be able to appreciate the patient detailed care and planning needed for radical treatment. The success of treatment will depend on the skill, accuracy and attention to detail of all concerned – technicians, radiographers, physicists and doctors.

Moulds for small-field beam-directed treatment are commonly used for lesions in head and neck, e.g. fauces, pituitary, antrum, larynx, and for some cases in the thorax, e.g. oesophagus. Since the patient wears the mould during actual treatment, there is no need to mark the skin itself. In others, e.g. breast, regional therapy in Hodgkin's disease and in palliative treatments, the treatment fields are outlined on the patient's skin with a dye, commonly gentian violet or a marking pencil. These serve the same purpose as a mould and enable the radiographer to position the fields accurately and in the same way at every session. They are put on with care and must not be removed. They tend to rub off through friction from clothing and bedding, aided by sweating. The marks may need reinforcing during the course of treatment, either in the treatment department or on the ward.

## Time and dose factors

In any radiation treatment there are always two fundamental factors to be decided:

1. *Dose* — what total dosage (in rads) should be given?
2. *Time* — how is this dose to be distributed in time? Should it be delivered in a 'single shot' or in fractions, and over what length of time?

These two factors are not independent of each other.

A dose of 2000 rads may suffice for a small (1 cm) skin cancer if delivered in a single treatment session, but if delivered in five daily fractions (5 × 400 rads) it would be insufficient. To achieve a comparable curative result, it would have to be 5 × 600 = 3000 rads. If we took two weeks — 10 treatment sessions — the dose would have to be 10 × 450 = 4500 rads. This is a general rule — the longer the overall time, the higher the dosage needed to achieve a comparable result.

It would of course be very convenient to use single shot treatments, but this is possible only for very small superficial lesions and even then the cosmetic results are liable to be inferior and the risk of necrosis higher. It was once thought that a single large dose was optimal for cancers generally, even in internal organs, but the unfortunate effects soon led to the use of smaller and smaller repeated doses over longer periods of time. This is the basis of modern technique — i.e. *protracted fractionation,* usually over several weeks.

This is superior both in safety and in curative effect. It is better tolerated by the tissues and takes advantage of the difference in radiosenstivity between cancerous and normal tissue. The sequence of events is pictured on Fig. 5.5. The cancer cells suffer progressive damage as the course proceeds and the gap between them and the normal cells widens. Eventually all the tumour cells are irreversibly damaged while normal cells can still recover. Figure 5.6 shows what occurs when dosage is too high or too low.

*Daily* treatments — Monday to Friday — are usual. This began as an administrative convenience, though there is no reason why it should remain the only method or the best method. Some centres now treat many cases three times a week — Monday, Wednesday, Friday. Results are equally good, possibly better in some lesions, and the strain on the patient is likely to be less.

*Split course.* This is another variation, e.g. a fortnight's treatment, after which the patient is rested for two to three weeks, then the treatment resumed for a further week or two; there may be a third course after a further rest. This is particularly useful for elderly patients. It imposes less strain on them and enables us to avoid troublesome radiation reactions,

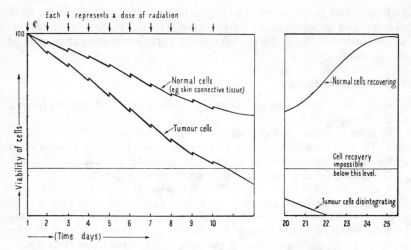

Fig. 5.5 Diagrammatic representation of a successful course of radiation treatment. For explanation see text.

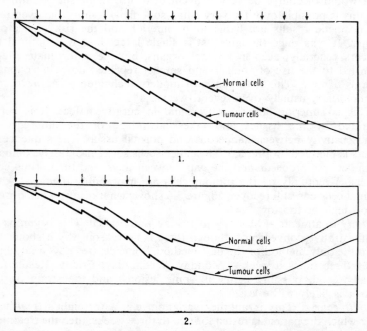

Fig. 5.6 Diagrammatic representation of unsuccessful courses of radiation treatment. (1) Course too long, resultant permanent injury to normal tissues and inability to heal. (2) Course too short, some tumour cells remain active to form later recurrence.

keep the treatment within tolerance limits, and often achieves better results than a standard course.

These technical questions of dosage and time are clearly of quite fundamental importance to the radiotherapist, as they may make all the difference between success and failure. We shall not attempt to go into further detail. The pros and cons rest on complex radiobiological considerations which are the subject of intensive recent research and there has in fact been a minor revolution in our thinking in the past decade. Nurses on radiotherapy wards are likely to hear much discussion among the medical staff on such topics, as there are no universally accepted treatment regimes. Different centres – and different radiotherapists even at the same centre – have different views on optimal regimes. It is of course possible to achieve successful results by more than one technique and judgement must be based on experience. At present there is a good deal of heart-searching among radiotherapists concerning the basis of their therapy and recent advances in radiobiological knowledge have called in question some of our traditional techniques. There is room for much experimentation with variations in time and dose patterns.

## Radiosensitivity of tumours

This is another factor of obviously fundamental importance. Tumours like normal tissues vary in their vulnerability to radiation and this depends chiefly on their rate of growth.

Table 5.1 lists some of the most important growths in the order of their radiosensitivity. It is a useful approximation, but there are exceptions, e.g. most lymphosarcomas melt away very rapidly, but the occasional case will prove unresponsive even to high dosage. Most cancers of rectum or melanomas are fairly insensitive, but a few prove to be sensitive.

Table 5.1 Tumour radiosensitivity

| | |
|---|---|
| *Highly sensitive* | |
| Reticuloses – e.g. lymphosarcoma, leukaemia, Hodgkin's | complete local disappearance to be expected |
| Seminoma of testis | |
| Medulloblastoma, neuroblastoma, nephroblastoma (Wilms) | |
| | |
| *Sensitive* | |
| Basal cell carcinoma | complete local disappearance to be expected |
| Epithelial carcinoma – skin, mouth, cervix, bladder etc. | |
| Carcinoma of breast | |
| Carcinoma of lung | |
| Carcinoma of ovary | |

*Poorly Sensitive*

| | |
|---|---|
| Sarcoma – osteosarcoma, fibro-sarcoma | complete local disappearance |
| Malignant melanoma (most cases) | possible, but not usually to be |
| Glioma | expected |
| Carcinoma of rectum | only temporary growth restraint |
| Carcinoma of kidney | usually to be expected |

The most important factor of all is the biological nature and behaviour of the particular cell type of the particular growth. Growths, like people, are never twice the same. Unexpected successes and failures occasionally occur for no apparent reason and there is no way at present of accurately assessing in advance the responsiveness of a particular tumour.

It is important to draw a distinction between *radiosensitivity* and *radiocurability*. For example, many of the highly sensitive group (e.g. lymphosarcoma), although responsive locally, are usually incurable as they tend either to produce distant secondaries at an early stage or to originate in several regions simultaneously or successively (multi-focal origin).

The highest proportion of successes is achieved in the epithelial cancers (especially squamous) of moderate sensitivity such as skin, mouth, cervix etc.

### Oxygen in radiotherapy

It is a fact of experience that tumours well supplied with blood vessels are more likely to respond to radiation than similar growths with poor blood supply. The difference seems to depend on the presence or absence of oxygen, which is normally carried in the red blood cells.

Growths tend to outstrip the available blood supply owing to cell multiplication and compression of vessels, with slowing of local circulation and partial necrosis which causes local oxygen lack. Thus the outer parts of a tumour may be well supplied with blood and oxygen, while the centre is deprived, i.e. relatively anoxic (Greek 'a(n)' = not).

Anoxic cells are only one-third as radiosensitive as fully oxygenated cells and these foci will tend to persist after the rest of the growth has responded and later give rise to recurrence.

*Hyperbaric oxygen therapy.* (Greek 'hyper' = excess, 'baros' = pressure). To counter this, additional oxygen can be supplied. During treatment the patient can inhale oxygen via a face mask from a cylinder alongside the treatment couch. This is not an efficient method and the effect of oxygen is best exploited by having the patient in a high-pressure tank, in which high oxygen concentration at about three times atmospheric pressure can be maintained during treatment.

Hyperbaric therapy is now under trial. It involves special technical difficulties and risks, but encouraging results have been claimed in advanced cases. If these are confirmed, we shall see the technique more widely used and improved results may be obtained in cases previously considered too advanced or too resistant for conventional radiotherapy.

## The treatment of choice

It will be useful to list the chief sites at which the various methods have been found to achieve the best results. The following classification (Tables 5.2-5.6) would not be universally accepted. In fact, no classification can hope to be since there are quite wide divergences in resources, experience and judgement. It should be taken as a broad generalisation with considerable room for flexibility.

*Hormones* are almost never the treatment of choice in the first instance. They are useful in selected cases of prostate, breast, thyroid, body of uterus, and kidney. (see Ch. 12).

Table 5.2 Surgery – The treatment of choice

---

Stomach, intestine, colon, rectum, pancreas, kidney, prostate
Wilms's tumour (in association with radiation and chemotherapy)
Bone – most primary tumours
Fibrosarcoma
Melanoma
Testis – orchidectomy for primary mass
Radiation may be useful for palliation (e.g. rectum) or pre-operatively (e.g. osteosarcoma)

---

Table 5.3 Radiation – The treatment of choice

---

Mouth – including lip, tongue, cheek, alveolus, fauces
Intra-nasal, accessory sinuses (antrum etc.), middle ear, naso-pharynx, oro-pharynx, hypopharynx
Skin – except melanoma
Uterus – cervix
Bladder – all except stage 1 growths
Larynx – vocal cords
Testis – seminoma (for secondaries)
Medulloblastoma – after surgical exploration
Lymphomas – Hodgkin's and others (cytotoxics very often useful as alternative, especially in late stages and leukaemias).

---

Table 5.4 Surgery – The first line

---

In operable cases, but radiation is justified even in early cases if surgery is contra-indicated. Useful results from palliative radiotherapy.

| | |
|---|---|
| Breast | Body of uterus |
| Lung | Ovary |
| Brain | Oesophagus |
| Urethra | Thyroid |
| Testis – teratoma (secondaries) | |
| Salivary glands (parotid etc.) | |
| Secondary carcinoma in lymph-nodes | |

---

Table 5.5 Radiation — The first line

Though results usually poor with any form of treatment.
Hypopharynx (epiglottis, piriform fossa, arytenoids)
Post-cricoid
Naso-pharynx
Neuroblastoma (in association with surgery and cytotoxics)


Table 5.6 Cytotoxic drugs — the treatment of choice

Acute leukaemia
Choriocarcinoma
Burkitt's lymphoma
For cytotoxic drugs as palliatives see Table 13.1 p. 222

# 6. Biological Effects of Radiation

*'Contrariwise', continued Tweedledee, 'if it was so, it might be; and if it were so, it would be; but as it isn't, it ain't. That's logic.'*
Lewis Carroll (Through the Looking Glass)

The diagnostic radiologist is interested in the photographic effect of the rays after differential absorption in tissues. The radiotherapist on the other hand is interested in their biological effect on living cells. As we have seen ionisation produces physico-chemical change. If the change involves important cell constituents, it will interfere with function, and the most important function from our standpoint is cellular reproduction – i.e. cell division by mitosis (pp. 10-11).

Interference with mitosis is usually the earliest visible effect, and is readily demonstrated both micrscopically and clinically. Figure 6.1 shows the visible effects of chromosome damage and this is the characteristic radiation effect in cells. There is no difference between normal and cancer cells in this respect.

The action of ionising radiation is always destructive, though the damage may be great or small. If small, the cell will recover and function normally (or almost so). If great, it will either die or be unable to reproduce – and this is enough to stop the cancerous process. It was once thought that the rays could have a stimulating effect, but this is not so and any apparent stimulation is an indirect effect due to inhibition of other cells.

The cellular effects may be summarised as follows:
                    1. Direct effects      2. Indirect effects

*1. Direct effects*

a. Some cells are killed outright. This is not usually very important and only affects certain rapidly growing cells.

b. Some cells die in attempted mitosis. This is the most important mechanism. There is no immediate visible effect on the cell at all, but when it goes into mitosis at a later stage, the damage will reveal itself (see Fig. 6.1) and the cell will break down and die. The time elapsing before this happens depends on the cell's rate of growth, which is the same thing as the doubling time (pp. 21-2). It may happen very soon – within a few hours – but it may not happen for days or weeks or even years, particularly in normal tissue.

c. Some cells are sterilised by premature 'ageing', so that they never attempt to go into mitosis and are thus made harmless.

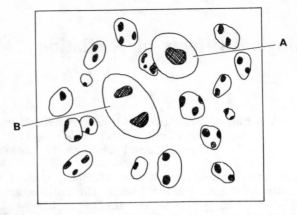

Fig. 6.1 (a) Microscopic appearance of rapidly-growing cancer, showing some cells in process of division (mitosis). A, mass of chromosomes in middle of cell at commencement of activity. B, the twin daughter masses have moved to opposite poles of the cell prior to actual division. (Compare Fig.2.1, p. 10).

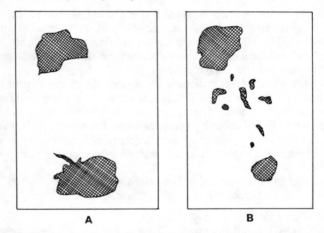

Fig. 6.1 (b) 'Close-ups' of the nuclei of tumour cells to show the effects of radiation. A, the daughter chromosome masses in the process of normal division. B, after radiation, showing the broken chromosome fragments left behind.

## 2. Indirect effects

a. Damage to local blood supply cuts off nutrition and causes local cell death.

b. Damaged cells fall victim to the tissue defence cells of the reticulo-endothelial system.

After destruction of the cancer cells, the wound is healed, just like any other type of wound, by reparative growth of normal tissue in the form of a scar. It is most important to appreciate that the tumour bed – fibrous tissue, blood vessels, epithelium etc. – plays a vital part in the final destruction and removal of a cancer and in the ultimate process of healing.

Consequently the dosage delivered to a growth must not be allowed to exceed the tolerance of these normal tissues, otherwise healing will not take place and the result will be a permanent necrosis. *The aim of the radiotherapist is to inflict the maximum damage on the cells of a cancer consistent with retaining the reparative powers of the surrounding normal tissues.*

*Radiosensitivity.* All living cells, normal or abnormal, can be damaged or destroyed by ionising radiation – if the dose absorbed is big enough. But the dose needed to produce comparable effects varies with the type of cell and tissue. For instance, the rapidly dividing parent cells of leucocytes in bone marrow will be seriously damaged by a dose which will have no obvious effect on the bone cells nearby whose rate of division is very slow indeed. This resistance or vulnerability is referred to as *sensitivity* of a tissue or growth and is clearly of fundamental importance in radiotherapy.

Radiotherapy is possible only because most cancers are more radiosenstive than their environment – i.e. they can be lethally damaged by a dose of radiation which will weaken but not kill the tumour bed. But if a growth consists of cells that are actually no more sensitive than their normal neighbours, then it cannot be satisfactorily treated by radiation since a cancericidal dose would at the same time prohibit healing.

When the cells of a cancer have been destroyed or sterilised by radiation, a tissue gap (e.g. an ulcerated surface) is left and this cellular wound acts as a growth-promoting stimulus, like any other kind of wound. Normal tissue controls can now come into play and fibrous tissue, blood vessels and epithelium can regenerate and proliferate until the gap is healed.

## Effects of radiation on normal tissues

*Radiosensitivity of different tissues*

There is a scale of sensitivity, from the highly sensitive to the relatively insensitive. The former are readily damaged by low doses of radiation, the latter can tolerate much larger doses (though not without sustaining some damage).

The *sensitive group* includes:

1. Reproductive cells of testis and ovary.
2. Cells in bone marrow and elsewhere that produce blood cells – i.e. haemopoietic tissue.
3. Epithelial lining of alimentary tract.
4. Epithelium of skin – i.e. epidermis.

*Intermediate sensitivity group:* Liver, kidney, many other glands – (thyroid, etc.).

*Low sensitivity group:* Muscle, bone, connective tissue, nerve tissue.

## The skin

This is a subject of prime importance since we are bound to irradiate the skin in most treatments, even if it is not the site of the tumour.

In superficial and deep therapy, the skin reaction is the limiting factor in dosage since the highest dose is on the actual skin surface and falls progressively in the deeper tissues (Figs. 4.14 and 4.15, p. 67). *Skin sensitivity* is taken as the 'yardstick' for measuring the sensitivity of other tissues. The characteristic radiation effect on skin is *erythema* (Greek for 'redness'), and in the days before definition of the roentgen and the rad, the 'erythema dose' was actually used as the measure of radiation dosage. In the orthovoltage (200 kV) era skin reactions were a very useful guide in actual treatment and could give warning signals to the therapist. Nowadays with the advent of megavoltage, which produces maximum dosage below the skin surface (Fig. 4.15, p. 67) skin reactions are not such limiting factors but are still of fundamental importance.

There is always an interval of time or *latent period* before a skin reaction appears, since it is an inflammatory reaction following the breakdown of damaged cells (basal cells of the epidermis which are the most actively growing cells of the skin). In a typical course of treatment, erythema begins in about two weeks.

### Radio-Dermatitis

This may be acute or chronic.

1. *Acute.* This occurs typically in patients undergoing a course of treatment and receiving a large dose in a short time.

2. *Chronic.* This includes late effects in:

a. patients − after months or years.

b. radiation workers (in industry etc.), or patients who receive small doses accumulating over a long period of time − usually many years − and do not pass through any acute phase.

The acute reaction may be divided into four stages or degrees of severity, with increasing dosage:

*First degree.* This is the *epilation dose* (Latin $e$ = out, *pilus* = hair) due to the destructive effect on hair roots. The hairs become loose and may be pulled out painlessly or fall out spontaneously. This happens about 18 days after an epilation dose and the hair grows again after 2-3 months. The effect was used in treatment of ringworm of the scalp, but has now given way to modern antibiotics.

*Second degree.* This is the typical bright-red erythema, sharply localised to the irradiated area. Sweat glands are inhibited and may be permanently destroyed. The hair will fall out; it usually grows again, but may not. When the erythema subsides, there is often some residual pigmentation, like sunburn, which may be permanent. There is usually some itching and some temporary dry peeling (*dry desquamation*) as the superficial horny layer of the epidermis becomes thickened and flaky and scales off (Latin *de* = off, *squama* = scale).

*Third degree.* The erythema is deeper and purplish. Blisters appear, raising the epidermis; these coalesce and burst, forming superficial ulcers exuding serum – i.e. *moist desquamation*. If left exposed, an adherent scab forms. Healing is usually rapid and complete in 2-3 weeks. Sweat glands are destroyed and loss of hair is permanent.

*Fourth degree.* The first three stages may be seen in normal treatment, but the fourth stage – the radiation *burn* or acute necrosis – should not normally be seen at all. It represents an overdose due to a technical mistake or an error of judgement. The erythema is intensely dark, blisters go deeper than the epidermis to involve the whole skin or even deeper, and the whole surface eventually sloughs off. Like an ordinary heat burn, it may be very painful. Healing may occur, but is always a long and doubtful matter of weeks or months, chiefly because of the destruction of blood vessels.

### Individual and local variations.

People vary in their sensitivity to ionising radiation, just as they do to ultra-violet rays (sunburn). Blondes with fair hair and fair skin are more sensitive than brunettes.

Different parts of the body vary also. The more sensitive areas include those subject to moisture and friction (axilla, groin, vulva, anus) and those with a relatively poor blood supply (back of hand, back and sole of foot, midline of back, and areas overlying bone or cartilage, e.g. pinna).

### Sequelae to skin reactions: Chronic radio-dermatitis

After treatment carried to high dosage, the skin will show some radiation effect for a long time, usually permanently, especially after superficial or deep therapy.

All the following changes are now seen far less frequently since the introduction of megavoltage with its skin-sparing effects (p. 68).

*Ischaemia.* Many of the late effects of therapeutic doses in the skin or any other organ are due to the destruction and choking of local blood vessels with consequent ischaemia, often associated with fibrosis. We shall have occasion to refer to this when discussing particular treatment, e.g. complications of radium treatment in cervical cancer (p. 134) and effects on brain, bone, bowel etc. (see below).

*Pigmentation.* This may vary from light to very dark brown and will show the size of the irradiated field. It may be distributed in a patchy manner, especially at the edges of a treated area, and may be mingled with whitish patches of depigmented atrophic skin.

*Atrophy.* After a moist desquamation, the ulceration heals by formation of a new epidermis growing in from the edges. This is never normal in colour or texture and may be markedly depigmented, a thin papery covering which is very liable to later breakdown on slight injury.

*Thickening.* The skin may heal with considerable fibrosis of the dermis, giving a typical leathery feel with loss of elasticity.

*Telangiectasia,* i.e. dilatation of terminal blood vessels (Greek 'tele' = distant; 'angion' = vessel; 'ectasia' = widening). Destruction or narrowing of the small arteries of the skin may lead to compensatory dilatation of capillaries, which can be very disfiguring.

*Late ulceration.* An atrophic area is always vulnerable to injuries that would normally be of negligible importance. A scratch or burn, even years later, may lead to a persistent breakdown. This is late necrosis; it is very slow to heal and may need excision and grafting.

*Malignancy.* This is a good example of the carcinogenic effect of chronic irritation (p. 13). In pioneer X-ray and radium workers, before the dangers were realised, skin changes appeared especially on the fingers. The skin became dry, lost its elasticity, and erythema formed round the nails, which became fissured and irregular and might be shed. Later warts and fissures appeared on the skin and eventually, after some years, epitheliomatous degeneration occurred.

Similar changes also happened in some patients subjected to repeated courses of radiation, especially for non-malignant conditions (pruritus, psoriasis etc. – see p. 246). These dangers are now well appreciated in industrial and medical situations, and are – or should be – chiefly of historical interest.

### Treatment of skin reactions

*Explanation to patients.* Patients should always be given a simple explanation of the likely effects of treatment on the skin – and any other organs likely to be affected such as bowel and bladder. It is useful to have a leaflet to hand out at the start, telling them what to expect and what precautions to take – Fig. 6.2 – otherwise reactions may cause needless alarm. If moist desquamation is expected, they should be told of the probable breakdown and discharge, crusting and eventual healing after two weeks or more. They should be assured that these are normal reactions, not 'burns'.

---

**INSTRUCTIONS TO PATIENTS
TREATED BY X-RAYS OR RADIUM**

**Care of the Skin**

Some redness and tenderness of the skin is to be expected about two to three weeks after beginning treatment.

It is important to observe the following instructions in order to keep the skin healthy and avoid trouble now or in the future:
1. Keep the area dry.
2. Do not wash the part (unless permitted by the doctor).
3. Do not apply ointments or lotions (unless prescribed by the doctor).
4. Do not apply hot fomentations, either during the treatment or afterwards.
5. Avoid direct sunshine or cold (winds, etc.) on the part.

---

Fig. 6.2 Pamphlet of instructions given to patients at the start of a course of treatment.

In the milder reactions, little or no special treatment may be necessary, e.g. in dry desquamation – unless the part is exposed to friction when a simple covering may be useful until the skin has healed. Even with a moist desquamation, if it is only a small area (e.g. a small epithelioma of the face), it is often quite satisfactory to leave it alone, allow it to crust over and leave healing to proceed until the crust drops off the new epidermis. If infection underneath the crust is suspected, it may be removed with forceps. If infection is present or threatens during the course of treatment, an antiseptic cream such as Hibitane or Cetavlex (cetrimide) can be used.

In first and second degree reactions, the chief complaint is usually of simple irritation or itching. An ordinary dusting or talcum powder may be used, but since most of these contain a heavy metal (zinc or bismuth) they should not be put on before treatment has finished, because the metal when irradiated gives rise to secondary radiation, which increases the skin dose and therefore the severity of the reaction. Instead a simple starch or baby powder should be used. For the same reason zinc oxide adhesive strapping should be avoided and sellotape or micropore used instead. In areas of friction, lanolin or tulle gras may be applied. When the full course of treatment is over, creams or ointments containing metals may be used freely, e.g. zinc and castor oil.

The patient should be cautioned against all forms of irritation to the treated area. It is usual to advise against washing the part at all until reactions are over. But it is not the (lukewarm) water or toilet soap that is to be feared, but the vigorous towelling likely to be applied after washing that really aggravates reactions. If the patient can be trusted, very gentle washing and gentle drying by dabbing are permissible.

If skin marks have been outlined on the patient for the radiographer's guidance, they must not be washed off. They tend to be removed by sweat and friction, and may need frequent reinforcing by marking pencil or gentian violet.

Shaving with ordinary razors is forbidden, as the trauma increases the severity of reactions. Electric shavers may be cautiously allowed. On the neck, tight or stiff collars should be discouraged because of chafing. Collars anyhow should be unbuttoned and a silk scarf makes an acceptable neckwear. Tight brassieres, corsets etc. are also bad as are counter--irritants like Thermogene wool.

In short all forms of irritation, mechanical, thermal or chemical – including hot water bottles – are to be avoided since they increase the severity of reactions, just as in sunburn.

Moist reactions usually need dressings. Non-adhesive siliconised dressings are useful, or Melolin (which is expensive). An antiseptic may be required to prevent infection, for sepsis will delay healing and worsen the cosmetic result. Every department has a favourite prescription. One is an antiseptic dye such as gentian violet (1 per cent aqueous); a single layer of gauze is applied to the surface and the dye is painted over it several times daily and allowed to dry. No attempt is made to remove it at subsequent paintings. It has a coagulant effect and forms a protective coat which is left on until it eventually separates from the healed surface. If frequent dressings are needed, an oily preparation is useful like acriflavine emulsion, or flavine and paraffin.

Patients are fond of applying Vaseline, but this tends to hinder discharges and promotes infection. If the moist area is large or the patient's condition poor, hospital care is advisable with nursing as for an ordinary burn.

Fourth degree reactions, i.e. acute necrosis, need similar but more prolonged treatment. For chronic ulcers Aserbine cream is useful. If ulceration persists, excision and possibly grafting may be needed.

At the end of the course of radiotherapy, if skin reactions are present or anticipated, the patient should always be told what he should do and not do. Gentle washing is usually allowable after two to three weeks with lukewarm water. No special attempt should be made to rub off the skin markings.

### Reactions on mucous membranes

The gastro-intestinal mucosa is more sensitive than the skin since it renews itself at an even faster rate. Cancericidal doses would usually involve intolerable ulceration, diarrhoea, bleeding etc. with high morbidity and even mortality. This is why the common cancers of stomach and colon are not treatable by radiation, and even palliative treatment is seldom rewarding.

Mucosal reactions are comparable to skin reactions, allowing for structural differences. Instead of hairs and sweat glands, mucous and salivary glands are inhibited. There is no horny layer to flake off, but at the stage of superficial ulceration (third degree) the exuded fluid coagulates and forms a whitish membrane composed of fibrin − the fibrinous (or membranous) reaction − which can be mistaken for thrush. This membrane becomes yellowish and gradually decreases in size as healing proceeds.

In the mouth and pharynx, these reactions may cause unpleasant dryness, loss of taste, sore throat and dysphagia. In the oesophagus, which is bound to be involved in the treatment of lung and mediastinum, there may be soreness, painful spasm and dysphagia.

In the bowel, when abdomen or pelvis is treated, there may be spasm and diarrhoea which can lead to dehydration, and also bleeding. When cancer of the cervix is treated, the rectum (immediately behind the vagina) receives a considerable dose and some degree of proctitis is usual with irritation, tenesmus, passage of mucus and possibly blood. In the bladder, reactions may cause dysuria with pain and frequency.

Late effects on mucosal surfaces may appear after weeks, months or years. There may be adhesions, fibrosis and stenosis, leading to obstruction. There may be ulceration, fistulae and bleeding. Surgical intervention may be needed for any of these. Another possibility is a malabsorption syndrome.

*Treatment of mucosal reactions.* As a prophylactic measure, dental treatment should be carried out where necessary in head and neck cases. If extractions are needed, radiation treatment should be delayed for dental sepsis will not only increase the patient's discomfort, but may even prejudice the success of radiotherapy. If teeth are in the high-dose area, they are bound to be affected and their vitality impaired. Subsequent decay is more difficult to deal with because of the impaired blood supply which is an inevitable effect of high radiation dosage. Later extractions can prove very troublesome and may be followed by osteomyelitis and even necrosis of the mandible, so that some therapists even advise prophylactic removal of healthy teeth, especially molars.

When mouth and throat are involved, the diet should be light. Foods of high calorie value (e.g. Complan) are helpful. Mouth washes should be used liberally to remove viscid secretions. When the reaction is at its height, generally towards the end of the course or soon after, eating may be painful. Aspirin mucilage or a local anaesthetic before meals (e.g. Mucaine) will help. Hot or spiced foods (vinegar, pickles etc.) should not be given. If possible smoking and alcohol should be stopped.

Bowel reactions are common and important in the treatment of abdominal and pelvic lesions. Drugs may be required to control vomiting, spasm or diarrhoea – chlorpromazine (Largactil), codeine phosphate, Probanthine, opiates etc. Reactions may set in early and may at times be so marked that treatment will have to be interrupted for a few days, or in extreme cases stopped entirely.

*Effects on blood-forming tissues*

Haemopoietic tissue – mainly bone marrow and lymphoid tissue – is highly radiosensitive. The most marked effects are on the parent cells of the leucocytes, lymphocytes and platelets. Red cells are much less radiosensitive, as their life-cycle is much longer – about four months, as compared with a day or less for most white cells.

In patients, the effect on the blood count is very variable. It depends on many factors, particularly the size of the area treated and the amount of bone marrow irradiated. There is a fall in total white cells – *leucopenia* – and in platelets – *thrombocytopenia* or thrombopenia – but red cells may hardly be affected at all. If only a very small part of the body is under treatment, the effect on the blood will be negligible and in superficial therapy, e.g. for skin cancer – we do not bother about blood counts. But the larger the field and the more penetrating the radiation, the greater will be the effect on haemopoietic tissue. During most courses of therapy, full blood counts are usually made weekly and often more frequently – sometimes even daily.

In really large field therapy, e.g. abdominal baths, the white cell and/or platelet counts may be the limiting factor. If counts drop too far it will be necessary to suspend treatment for a few days (or even stop it completely), otherwise the patient will be dangerously exposed to infection because of leucopenia and haemorrhage because of thrombopenia. As to the lower limit of safety this is a matter of medical judgement and will vary from case to case. As a rough guide we may say that counts of less than 2000 white cells or 80 000 platelets (normal = 250 000 per cubic mm) are danger signals.

Just as for skin effects, marrow damage occurred in pioneer radiation workers who developed aplastic anaemia or even leukaemia as a result. This is another example of the carcinogenic effect of chronic irritation.

*Effects on reproductive organs*

The gonads (ovary and testis) contain two separate types of tissue:

a. Reproductive, for formation of germ cells (ova and sperm). They are among the most radiosensitive in the body.

b. Endocrine, for production of sex hormones (oestrogens and androgens).

*Males.* Sperm production can be temporarily halted by quite low doses, e.g. 50 rads. Permanent sterility occurs after about 1000 rads. Androgenic hormone production is much more radioresistant and this effect is rarely of clinical importance.

*Females.* Sterility can similarly be induced by radiation and depends on physiological age. Hormonal effects are more obvious and of much greater clinical importance than those in the male. Production of ovarian hormone can be reduced or abolished with temporary or permanent suppression of menstruation. This effect is used in inducing an artificial menopause (p. 247).

*Gene mutations* (see p. 107). Very low doses of radiation, too low to have any obvious effect on mitosis, can still affect the genes from which chromosomes are made and so produce genetic effects in the offspring. These mutations (Latin for 'changes') are almost always detrimental. Once produced they are permanent and transmitted to any offspring. When we treat the pelvis of a pre-menopausal patient to high dosage, e.g. for cancer of cervix, sterility will be inevitable and there will be no problem of gene mutations, since there will be no further children. In any event, the alternative surgical treatment would achieve the same result. But irradiation of the gonads, male or female, in the younger age group is only justified for life-saving purposes or for deliberately producing sterility, as in the artificial menopause.

Years ago, ovarian radiation at low dosage was used, e.g. for treatment of dysmenorrhoea or sterility. This would be frowned on today, as it would mean inevitable 'contamination of the stream of human life', even though the results might not be apparent until later generations. Genetic damage was vividly illustrated by the after-affects of the atomic bomb (pp. 14, 109).

*Radiation in pregnancy.* This is particularly, undesirable. Damage may be done either to the mother's ovaries or to the fetus. Gene mutations in the ovarian germ cells (ova) may cause changes in later children of the mother or in later generations. The fetus itself is highly vulnerable – not surprisingly, in view of the relatively enormous growth rate and the extreme immaturity of all its tissues. The first three months are the most dangerous, and even low dose radiation then can produce such defects as hare lip, cleft palate, mental deficiency, etc. Larger doses will kill the fetus and lead to abortion.

We now have evidence that fetal irradiation carries a definite risk of childhood leukaemia. Because of this, diagnostic X-ray departments, before taking films of the pelvis etc., enquire routinely into the menstrual history, to avoid exposure in women of reproductive age if there is a possibility of pregnancy.

*Effects on other organs*

Every organ in the body is affected to a greater or lesser extent, i.e. they have varying radiosensitivities. This is largely a function of growth rate, e.g. mature nerve cells never divide, so radiation damage does not show itself, whereas the stem cells of the blood are in continual active growth.

*Eye.* The conjunctiva is rather more sensitive than the skin, but most of the eye is relatively insensitive. Damage to the cornea, especially if accompanied by infection, can lead to corneal opacities with some degree of blindness. The lens is very liable to post-radiation changes – typically a few years after treatment. A dose of about 750-1000 rads can cause *cataract,* depending on the patient's age.

The lacrimal ducts, which begin at the inner ends of the eyelids, are at risk when lesions such as rodent ulcers of the inner canthus are treated. The radiation reaction in the duct can lead to blockage and if the obstruction is not relieved, it may be permanent. Tears will then be unable to escape by their normal channel to the back of the nose and will overflow on to the cheek (epiphora). To avoid this, it is good practice to send the patient to the eye department after the height of the reaction is over, for the duct to be syringed once or twice. This ensures its patency.

When treating cancers near the eye, e.g. nasal cavity, antrum, naso-pharynx – we try to minimise the dosage to the eye itself by specially arranged radiation fields and lead protection. But in some cases, e.g. a growth that has invaded the orbit, it is essential to include all or most of the eye in the high-dose region and we must accept the consequences if curative treatment is our aim. With megavoltage, the surface-sparing effect is valuable in lessening the actual dose which conjunctiva and cornea receive, and hence the severity of the inevitable conjunctivitis. When the reaction begins, antiseptic eye-drops or ointment should be used freely, e.g. sulphacetamide (Albucid) or hydrocortisone-neomycin.

Apart from cataract, degeneration of the globe is liable to occur at high dosage, with complete loss of vision. The eye will be painful and may have to be enucleated. This may occur about three years after radical dosage.

See also p. 161 for precautions taken in treatment of the eyelid.

*Kidney.* Radiation can damage renal blood vessels and lead to degenerative changes. The possible consequences are increased blood pressure (benign or malignant hypertension), and acute or chronic nephritis with raised blood urea, renal failure and uraemia.

The borderline of safety is about 2000 rads, and if the kidneys are included in the radiation field (e.g. in an abdominal bath) they must be shielded by lead blocks when this dose is reached, after being localised either by a plain X-ray film of the abdomen or by I.V.P.

*Brain and nerve tissue.* Although relatively resistant, serious effects can follow high dosage. This is due to damage to the blood supply of the brain or spinal cord, which in turn leads to degenerative changes. After treatment of a brain tumour, there may be late symptoms suggestive of recurrence, but these may be due to radiation damage alone. In the spinal cord, radiation myelitis can cause paralysis etc. even years later and be mistakenly attributed to metastasis.

When treatments are planned, e.g. to pharynx, oesophagus etc., see pp. 75-6 — we always take account of the dose to the central nervous system to ensure that tolerance is not exceeded.

*Bone and cartilage.* High dosage may result in devitalisation, necrosis (early or late), and fracture. Vascular damage is again the chief cause. In rare cases, malignant change (osteosarcoma or fibrosarcoma) has developed years afterwards. In growing bone, damage to the epiphysis can retard growth and cause, e.g. shortening of a limb or spinal scoliosis. This must be remembered whenever radiation is used in children.

Cartilage necrosis can occur in, e.g. the outer ear (pinna and external auditory meatus), nose (ala nasi) and larynx.

All these changes are aggravated, or precipitated by trauma and infection. Dental caries is an example we have already discussed.

*Lungs.* The inflammatory reaction in lung tissue — radiation pneumonitis — may cause serious scarring (fibrosis) which prevents the lung expanding properly and so reduces vital capacity and makes the patient more liable to pulmonary infection. We therefore try to avoid lung tissue. For example, in treating the chest wall in breast cancer, special techniques are used to minimise damage to underlying lung (Fig. 8.5, p. 121).

## Radiation sickness

This is a general reaction which is liable to occur during a course of treatment. Its severity depends on the part of the body and the volume of tissue which is irradiated. If we treat a small epithelioma on the skin, there will be no general reaction at all. But if we use large-field or 'bath' type of therapy for a deep tumour, especially if the upper abdomen is included, there may be marked general upset.

The clinical picture resembles sea-sickness – tiredness and weakness, headache and nausea, maybe vomiting. In very sensitive or debilitated patients there may be prostration and treatment may have to be interrupted.

The cause of radiation sickness is obscure. Radiation has a destructive effect on tissue, especially rapidly dividing cells. Abnormal breakdown products may act as toxic foreign protein, which the body is not accustomed to deal with, and cause a minor or major degree of shock. The nervous type of patient is more liable to sickness than the stoic and much good can be done by simple explanation before the course begins, with reassurance that some degree of tiredness etc. is to be expected and is not abnormal.

If drugs are indicated, a simple sedative may be enough or Vitamin $B_6$ (pyridoxin). There is no specific treatment for the sickness, but anti-sickness drugs may help, e.g. Avomine, Stemetil, Fentazine, chlorpromazine (Largactil). Adequate fluid intake should be maintained – 4-5 pints daily – to dilute and eliminate any offending toxins.

Radiation sickness is much less common than it used to be. This is due to better patient care, improved radiation techniques, and megavoltage (p. 68).

**Acute radiation syndrome** – this is described on p. 108-9.

# 7. Radiation Hazards and Protection

*To wilful men,*
*The injuries that they themselves procure*
*Must be their schoolmasters.*

Shakespeare (King Lear)

Since the effects of ionising radiation on living cells are harmful, protection of all workers exposed to them is an important matter. In the early days, the dangers were not known – especially the effects of repeated low-dosage exposure which might not appear until many years later. These had to be learned from painful experience, including fatalities. Today they are very well known and there is a complete organisation to guard against them.

The chief injuries possible in hospitals are those to (a) skin; (b) blood-forming organs; (c) gonads (genetic effects), and these have been discussed in Chapter 6.

The safety rules, together with elementary knowledge and common sense should remove all danger of injury to nurses and other hospital staff and there should be no more reason to fear the hazards of radiation than those of electrical equipment and fire.

## Protection regulations

Control of radiation hazards in the National Health Service is guided by an official *Code of Practice for the Protection of Persons against Ionising Radiation arising from Medical and Dental Use.* Behind this is the Medical Research Council's Committee on Protection, and also an important body of experts, the International Commission on Radiological Protection which studies all new knowledge and experience as it becomes available and suggests modifications in the dose levels considered to be safe.

There is an excellent booklet, *A Handbook for Nurses on the Safe Use of Ionising Radiations* published by Her Majesty's Stationery Office, which every nurse concerned with radiation work should read and own.

*Responsibility for safety.* The head of a department carries the day-to-day responsibility for the work and safety of his department. He shares this responsibility with several officers, all of whom work under the Controlling Authority of the hospital. This may be the Hospital Management Committee or Board of Governors:

1. *Radiological Protection Adviser* – a qualified physicist.

2. *Supervisory Medical Officer* – concerned with preliminary and later medical examinations to ensure the health of workers in the department.

3. *Radiological Safety Officers* – normally permanent members of the department, often senior radiographers or ward sisters, who have day--to-day responsibility of seeing that protection rules are observed.

There is also a *Radiological Protection Committee* to review local procedures, draw up Local Rules taking particular local circumstances into account – these are bound to vary somewhat from one institution to another – receive reports from the various officers and advise the Controlling Authority.

## Maximum permissible dose

The *Code of Practice* specifies maximum permissible dose levels for workers in radiological departments or with some contact with these departments. It is a rather complicated and technical matter and it is not necessary for us to go into full detail here. Doses are specified in rems, but for our purposes the rem may be regarded as equivalent to the rad.

There are two groups to consider:

1. Designated persons.    2. Other staff.

1. *Designated persons* are those whose work involves exposure to such an extent that the maximum permissible dose might in some circumstances be approached. Normally this dose is never expected to be reached, but if there is even the possibility due to accident, then the staff involved are *designated*. They include radiographers, radium curators, physicists, doctors and nurses on radiotherapy wards.

2. *Other staff* are persons not directly involved with ionising radiations, but who may come into contact with it in the course of their normal duties, e.g. porters, maintenance workers, cleaners, etc.

*Maximum permissible* dose is that dose which, in the light of present knowledge, is not expected to cause appreciable bodily injury to a person at any time during her/his lifetime.

The current maximum permissible dose for whole-body exposure is 3 rems per calendar quarter (i.e. 13 weeks) or 5 rems in a year, and a cumulative dose of about 200 rems in the whole of working life. The average dose should therefore be kept below 0.1 rem to the whole body per week. If only the extremities are exposed, e.g. hands – higher doses are allowable.

The limit of 3 rems a quarter does not apply to abdominal exposure of women of reproductive age, which should not exceed 1.3 rems in a 13-week period.

## Radiation monitoring

To measure the doses actually received by individual staff during working hours, nurses and other members of the hospital wear a small plastic holder or cassette, about 4 × 3 cm, usually pinned to clothing at chest or waist level. This 'badge' contains a piece of X-ray film, and any radiation reaching it will produce a certain amount of blackening when the film is developed. The degree of blackening can be read by a special instrument and gives a measure of the amount of radiation that caused it. The badge must be worn continuously, i.e. all the time that radiation exposure is possible, and for theatre work it must be transferred from normal clothing to theatre garments.

The Radiological Safety Officer changes the film at intervals – e.g. every month or week depending on the type of work, and records the measured doses of each person. These dose records are preserved, and if a person leaves one department or institution to take up work in another, her dose record is transferred.

There is now a standard international symbol (Fig. 7.1) to denote the presence of ionising radiation – actual or potential. It is black on a yellow background and is displayed on all doors leading into rooms which house X-ray machines, radium or other radioactive sources; also on the beds of patients carrying such sources during treatment.

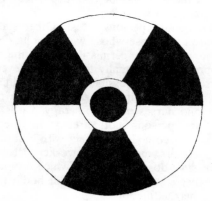

Fig. 7.1 The international symbol denoting the presence – actual or potential – of ionising radiation. Black on yellow background.

### Protection in X-ray therapy departments

Ward nurses, unlike radiographers, will have little direct contact with X-ray or gamma ray therapy units. Protection here is relatively simple. The walls, doors etc., of the rooms housing the machines, incorporate adequate thicknesses of lead or special concrete so that only negligible doses can escape. With megavoltage, adequately absorptive doors become so heavy that they are often replaced by a simple form of maze.

The patient is alone in the treatment room during actual treatment, but is under continuous observation. For low or medium voltage equipment, observation is through a lead-glass window in the wall. For megavoltage, a periscopic system of mirrors is sometimes used or else a television camera. The patient should be able to communicate with the radiographer at the control desk in case of emergency or distress – if necessary, by a microphone arrangement.

X-ray machines are switched on and off, like electric lights, and when switched off give out no radiation at all. Gamma ray beam units (cobalt, caesium etc.) cannot be switched off in this way since the radioactive source emits rays continuously. But at the end of a treatment, either the beam is cut off by closing a shutter or the source is moved mechanically to a safe position inside a large mass of metal which absorbs almost all the radiation. It is then quite safe to enter the treatment room, but it is common sense to stay there no longer than necessary.

Machines – except for superficial X-rays – are automatically switched off when the door of the treatment room is opened. This is to prevent accidental exposure of staff. In the case of some low-voltage machines used for skin therapy ('contact' therapy or Grenz rays) essential staff may remain in the treatment room. With one model, the therapist may actually hold the tube by hand during treatment, but full use is made of protective lead-rubber gloves and aprons and lead glass screens.

## Protection from small sealed radioactive sources

These include radium, cobalt, caesium, gold etc. used for their gamma rays, and also beta-ray emitters such as strontium-90. Radium presents the greatest problems of all as its gamma rays are very penetrating and it gives off a radioactive gas (radon) which will leak through a damaged container. The containers must be handled at some stage, either for insertion in the body or for threading, cleaning and preparing them for application to patients. The person involved usually has to work close to the radioactive source.

There are three fundamental methods of reducing radiation hazards and doses to personnel:

1. Distance. 2. Shielding. 3. Speed.

1. *Distance*. The farther one is from a source, the smaller the dose received in a given time – in accordance with the inverse square law – Fig. 7.2.

2. *Shielding*. Thick slabs of dense material such as lead can absorb most of the radiation.

3. *Speed*. The shorter the time spent near a source, the lower the dose received.

Radium containers have to be manipulated in the storage room, preparation room, operating theatre and wards, as well as transported between storage and operation sites. Remote handling equipment, to increase the distance between worker and source, and automatic devices to reduce the time in manipulation, are used as much as possible.

Radioactive sources are never touched by hand; long-handled forceps

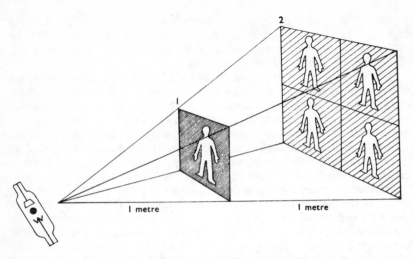

Fig. 7.2 Inverse Square Law, showing the importance of distance. If distance is doubled, intensity diminishes not to $\frac{1}{2}$ but to $\frac{1}{2}^2 = \frac{1}{4}$. If distance is trebled intensity $= \frac{1}{3}^2 = 1/9$, and so on. (*Courtesy Mr. J. O. Robinson and Dr. A. Jones, Surgery, Longmans*).

are always employed to keep them as far as possible from the body and fingers. Full use is made of lead screening, at least 2 in (= 5 cm) thickness, and simple L-pieces (Fig. 7.3).

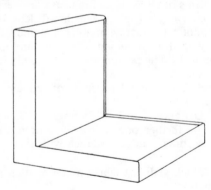

Fig. 7.3 Lead L-piece for protection from gamma rays.

*Threading* of needles before their use in the theatre can involve considerable exposure of the fingers. This is minimised by a special lead block in which the needles can be embedded with only the eye projecting (Fig. 7.4). A needle threader consisting of a simple wire loop which passes easily through the eye of the container saves time (Fig. 8.16, p. 140).

*Sterilisation* of containers must be done in a lead shielded steriliser. It must never be allowed to boil dry, otherwise overheating might lead to a burst needle or tube. Boiling is now being superseded by chemical sterilisation, e.g. ethylene oxide – which avoids this risk.

*Cleaning* of containers is a tiresome but necessary procedure. It can now be done by ultrasonic rays after immersion in a suitable fluid.

*Storage* of large quantities of radium etc. requires a safe containing a large mass of lead with drawers in the middle.

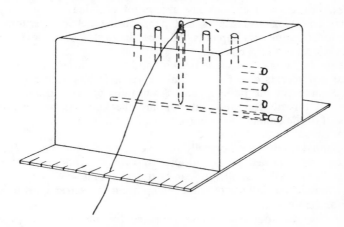

Fig. 7.4 Lead block for holding radium needles for threading.

*Transport* about the hospital requires shielded carriers – a lead-lined box with a long handle – or better still a special trolley on wheels with 1 inch lead shielding. This gives a good reduction of radiation dose without making the trolley too heavy to handle.

In modern departments, transport problems and exposure can be eased considerably by sensible arrangement of rooms, e.g. lift communication between ward and radium room, and preparation room next to the theatre with direct access through the wall.

*The care of radium.* Precautions are necessary to safeguard radium containers, not just because of their high cost, but because of the potential danger if they are lost.

Adequate records for the movements of radium to and from the safe are essential. It is usual for the radium to be in the direct charge of a curator or custodian, or a senior nurse or radiographer. Whenever sources are required for treatment the person responsible will check them and sign for them. There must be a strict system for keeping track of sealed sources in use, and the person responsible for them must be known.

*Sealed sources in the ward.* The commonest situations are tubes in the uterus and vagina and needles in the tongue. Some departments use surface moulds frequently and these patients will also be on the ward, preferably in side-wards. Otherwise they must be distributed as widely as possible. Beds should be at least 8 ft from adjacent beds, centre to centre, and should carry a notice to show the presence of radioactive sources (Fig. 7.1) with details of their number and strength.

Some hospitals have mobile lead screens, positioned at the sides and foot of the bed to protect the nurse's body and reduce exposure during nursing procedures – toilet, dressings, checking insertions and removing sources. Particular occasions are change of dressing over an implant, catheter emptying and use of bed pans during pelvic insertions, and mouth toilet during oral implants. All procedures should be carried out as rapidly as reasonably possible.

Needle implants (e.g. tongue or skin) and vaginal inserts should be examined at intervals of 4-6 hr to make sure there has been no displacement. Sources in the patient cannot normally be seen, though the attached silk threads can, and counting and checking can be done by this means. If dislodgement has occurred – e.g. needle end showing – medical help must be obtained at once.

Implanted needles are normally removed by a doctor. The needles are counted and returned in a lead-lined box to the radium store room. Removal of a surface applicator can be done by a nurse who should wear gloves, handle it as little as possible, and place it in the transport holder at once for removal.

Utero-vaginal sources are also removed by the nurse. If there is a vaginal pack, this is dealt with first, then the vaginal applicators, and finally the intra-uterine tube. Gloves and aseptic technique should be used, as well as long-handled forceps – *the sources themselves should never be touched by hand*. The nurse should keep as far away from the radium as possible and keep the lead screen, if present, between herself and the sources. After counting and checking, they are returned to the store.

*Loss of sealed sources.* Loss of radium on the ward is always a potential hazard. Patients carrying sources should not be allowed to leave the bed, or at least move outside a limited area. They must certainly not be permitted to go to a toilet.

Counts of needles, tubes, etc. are made as a routine on removal from a patient. They are checked against the treatment record and any discrepancy dealt with at once. The thread of a needle may break, leaving the needle in the tissue – this can be checked by X-ray examination. Whenever a loss is suspected, it should be reported to physicist, sister, doctor and radiological safety officer. The patient should not be moved – nor should the dressings, bedding, furniture (bed-table, locker etc.) until the physicist has made an instrumental check. This is often a simple matter, with the aid of a portable battery-operated radiation detector.

In some wards dressings etc., are routinely tested in this way. In any case, they must not be destroyed until all sources have been accounted for. There may be a sensitive instrument permanently mounted at the door of the ward, which will give a warning signal — by light and sound — if a gamma ray source passes through.

Clearly a nurse should be conscious of the importance of strict counting and precise knowledge and control of the whereabouts and movements of all sources until responsibility passes from her to another person (radium curator etc.).

Conditions in different hospitals are variable and the Local Rules with which the nurse must be familiar are designed to take these conditions into account and should be followed faithfully in any emergency.

*Sources in the operating theatre.* In theatres and other rooms where sources are applied to patients, all practicable physical protection should be given, such as lead barriers mounted on wheels, boxes, L-pieces (Fig. 7.3) etc. Sources should remain behind these barriers as long as possible and be removed individually as required. Full use must be made of long-handled forceps and sources must be held as far from the nurse's body as practicable.

The commonest procedure in most hospitals will be utero-vaginal intracavitary insertions. Less common nowadays are needle implants, mostly in the mouth. Unsealed sources may also be inserted, e.g. radioactive gold or yttrium into abdominal or pleural cavity.

Nurses should receive thorough training in theatre routine with regard to radiation hazards, e.g. the safest place to stand when watching insertions, use of lead shields etc., importance of speed in handling and so on.

If a nurse accompanies a trolley with a patient containing radioactive sources back to the ward or X-ray diagnostic department, she should not walk at the side but at the head or foot, so as to increase the distance between herself and the sources.

*Unsealed sources* (see p. 53). These are always in liquid form. Apart from those in tracer studies, the only ones in common hospital use are: Iodine (I-131, by far the commonest); Phosphorus (P-32); Gold (Au-198); Yttrium (Y-90).

| | |
|---|---|
| I-131<br>Au-198 | emit beta rays and also penetrating gammas. All protection principles important — shielding, distance, speed of handling. |
| P-32<br>Y-90 | emit betas only, which do not generally pass through container wall. Simple shielding adequate, distance not so important. |

The same radiation hazards apply to unsealed as to sealed sources, but in addition there is the important risk of *contamination*. This risk cannot arise with sealed sources except in the rare event of a burst or leak in the metal container. Contamination may be:

a. *external* — on skin, bedding, furniture etc.;

b. *internal,* e.g. if the source gets into the mouth from the hands or is inhaled as dust.

In isotope departments or any place where unsealed sources are used, smoking, drinking and applying cosmetics are prohibited.

Patients should be in special side-wards if possible, with smooth walls and rounded corners for easy cleaning. Most of the principles given above for sealed sources can be applied to unsealed. The Local Rules will deal with modifications. The following are general points:

1. Wearing of gloves, aprons, and sometimes masks, caps and boots, e.g. for cleaning the room after a spill.

2. Special care with contaminated urine or vomit. Faeces are rarely contaminated enough to be a hazard.

3. Separate crockery and cutlery – preferably of a different colour.

4. Separate laundering of contaminated linen.

5. Separate toilets for patients, also separate bottles and bed-pans.

The most important unsealed isotope on the ward is radioactive iodine, and further precautions are given on p. 196.

*Accidental spills* of radioactive fluids may occur – e.g. a urine bottle when a patient has had a large therapeutic dose of iodine-131. So an emergency kit should always be kept on or near the ward, containing such items as – gowns, rubber gloves, swabs, long-handled forceps, mopping cloths and blotting paper, polythene sheeting with filter paper on one side, polythene bags, warning labels. The physicist and other officers should be informed. Contamination may involve the patient, the bed, floor, furniture, even the clothing of the nursing staff. Surfaces should be mopped until dry, and mopping material and forceps put into plastic bags. The area should then be covered with plastic sheeting which is then secured by adhesive tape. If possible, special boots should be worn and care taken to avoid spread of contamination by footwear.

*Visitors* are, of course, also exposed to radiation when near a patient and should be advised not to be too close for too long. Youngsters under six years of age, and pregnant women, should not be admitted because of the special hazard to growing tissues.

*Death* of a patient may occur while he is still carrying significant isotope burdens. Radium inserts etc., must be removed by a doctor. If the isotope cannot be removed, e.g. intracavitary radio-gold – the physicist must be informed and a special label attached to the body before it is sent to the mortuary. The mortuary attendant must also be told and he will see to it that the special precautions laid down for these emergencies are set in motion.

*Training* of all staff exposed to radiation is most important. They should receive theoretical and practical instruction and be familiar with the Local Rules so that they are in no doubt what to do either in routine or in emergencies. Rotation of staff nursing patients who carry radioactive sources is a commonsense measure to reduce exposure to individuals.

### Radiation hazards in peace and war

In the light of our knowledge about the biological effects of ionising radiation, we will now view the subject in a wider context. Radiotherapy is only a very minor source of radiation to mankind as a whole. We are all exposed to radiation from sources both natural and man-made.

*Natural sources* of ionising radiation are: (a) cosmic rays and (b) naturally occurring radioactive elements on the earth.

a. *Cosmic radiation* bombarding the earth from outer space includes electrons, neutrons and other particles. Most of it is filtered off by the earth's atmosphere, but the small fraction which gets by is highly penetrating and irradiates the whole body uniformly.

b. *Terrestrial radiation* comes from radioactive chemical elements which are distributed over most of the earth in minute quanitites in rocks and soils, especially granite rock. From these, gamma rays arise so that building bricks and stone are liable to be sources of radiation. Radon gas diffuses from the earth into the atmosphere where it is normally present in extremely low concentration. The normal human body itself contains traces of radioactive carbon and potassium as well as radium etc., absorbed from food and water and deposited in bone.

In considering the effects of natural radiation on mankind, our first concern must be the dose to the gonads. The average dose from all the above sources has been estimated at roughly 0.1 rad per year, or about 3 rads per generation of 30 years.

*Genetic effects.* Gene mutations have been mentioned on p. 94. Biologically they are of fundamental importance, as they provide the 'raw material' on which the evolutionary processes of natural selection can work. Mutations occur naturally and continually in genes at a definite but very low rate.

All genes are subject to possible mutations, but the causes are not clear. Genes are complex molecules and structural disturbances can arise from random chemical influences as well as ionising radiation. Natural background is responsible for only a fraction of ordinary mutations – perhaps 10 per cent. There is no reason to think that radiation, natural or otherwise, produces any novel type of change – its effect is simply to increase the rate or *frequency of mutation.*

Since the biological effects of gene mutations are generally harmful, the consequences are serious. They may be apparent as congenital abnormalities in the next generation or may not appear for several generations. Note that there are no serious consequences for the individual originally irradiated, only for his/her descendants. They are therefore of no importance if that individual cannot or does not have children.

*Man-made sources of ionising radiation.* These include the increasing uses of radiation in industry and medicine. *In medicine,* diagnostic X-rays contribute a far greater dose to the population as a whole than radiotherapy. *In industry,* radiography is widely used for e.g., examination of castings. Physicists, chemists, engineers, and others engaged in the production of X-ray tubes or radioactive isotopes are similarly exposed. Isotopes are employed in a wide variety of industrial processes for calibration, accurate control etc. The development of *atomic energy* plants has added a new sector on the industrial front and here radiation hazards involve many thousands of workers.

There are many *historic* examples of the dangers involved and some have already been described – skin cancers in pioneer X-ray and radium workers (p. 90), anaemia and leukaemia (p. 94), sterility (p. 94), cataract (p. 95) after some industrial accidents, bone sarcoma in luminous dial painters (p. 14), lung cancers in miners of radioactive ores.

### The acute radiation syndrome

This is exemplified by the *atom bomb.* At Hiroshima and Nagasaki, where the bombs fell in 1945, most of the casualties were due to blast and fire, but 15-20 per cent were from gamma and neutron radiation. The effective range for serious injury from radiation was about one mile, compared with three miles for flash burns and five miles for blast.

The radiation doses have been estimated and the survivors carefully followed up and observed. Other episodes have been: unintentional exposure in the Marshall Islands in the Pacific in 1954 in the course of bomb testing, affecting nearly 300 people; over a dozen accidents involving high exposure in industrial plants, laboratories and hospitals. All these plus experimental animal work, have given us a detailed picture of the effects and mechanisms of acute radiation damage.

1. Doses of about 700 rads – i.e. to the whole body at once – leave few if any survivors.

2. Doses of 450 rads make all victims very ill, and 50 per cent die in 2-3 months.

3. 150 rads cause illness in about half.

4. 100 rads cause sickness in about one-seventh, with very few deaths.

5. 50 rads rarely cause sickness.

The effects may be summarised under three headings:

(1) the *haematological syndrome;* (2) the *gastro-intestinal syndrome,* (3) the *central nervous system* (CNS) *syndrome.*

The typical sequence of events after a dose of about 400 rads is as follows. Nausea and vomiting within the first few hours, then a latent period of several days. Then sickness again, fever and weight loss. Intestinal ulceration now dominates the picture with diarrhoea, fluid loss, dehydration and prostration. Bleeding occurs from bowels, nose etc. Deaths begin in the third week, till 50 per cent succumb by the end of the third month. The rest recover very slowly and suffer premature ageing later and increased risk of cataract, leukaemia, amenorrhoea, sterility, etc.

At this level the chief target tissue is the bone marrow, where the parent cells of the peripheal blood cells are inhibited or killed. Lymphocytes are affected most, then the other white cells, then the megakaryocytes (from which platelets are derived). The red cell precursors are also sensitive, but since the life-span of the adult red cell is about four months, anaemia sets in later then leucopenia. Thrombopenia leads to haemorrhages, leucopenia to bacterial infection, especially from the bowel.

There is some direct effect on gastro-intestinal mucosa which is one of the fastest-growing tissues in the body and normally renews itself every two days. This is slowed down or prevented, with resultant ulceration and bacterial invasion leading to septicaemia.

At higher dose levels, over 1000 rads, the gastro-intestinal effect becomes even more important, with death in a few days from fluid loss and massive bacterial damage.

At above 2000 rads the CNS syndrome sets in, with headache, coma and convulsion. It is always fatal.

In those who survived the bomb a special hazard involved pregnant women. Abortions and stillbirths (i.e. birth of dead babies) were brought about. If the child in the womb survived, its brain development was liable to be retarded and it might be born with an abnormally small head and mental deficiency.

## Late hazards of atom bombs

The newer (thermoneuclear) bombs are thousands of times as powerful. In addition to the late hazards already mentioned (ageing, leukaemia, etc.) there are special dangers from the 'fall-out'. This is the radioactive dust containing fission products carried to great heights in the atmosphere with the vaporized material from the bomb. The fine particles are carried in air currents, settling down gradually to earth. These dust clouds can travel enormous distances, even encircling the earth many times over, so that *no part of the world is immune.* A bomb exploded e.g. in Nevada (U.S.A.) produces fall-out detectable in England after about five days. If the firing of test bombs continues at its present rate, the gonad dose involved will be quite low, only about 1 per cent of the natural background; but any marked increase in the number of bombs could soon become significant genetically to the future world population. As it is, the fall-out from a bomb can have fatal effects over an area of 7000 square miles and be dangerous for tens of thousands of square miles.

A special danger from fall-out concerns radioactive strontium, a fission product. This is soluble and is absorbed by plants, cattle, etc., and thereby reaches humans in food and drink. It behaves chemically like calcium and is deposited in bone tissue after absorption. It is therefore potentially capable of producing late effects comparable to those in the luminous-dial painters mentioned above. So far the danger is negligible but is one of the indices that have to be watched.

Taking all the man-made sources together (radiography, industry, bombs, etc.) the total gonad dose is estimated to amount to about 20 per cent of the natural background, or rather less than 1 rad in a generation of 30 years. This is a figure that need cause no present alarm. Constant watch is now kept on the dosage to the population from industry, atomic energy plants, fall-out, etc., and our knowledge of the potential hazards is extensive enough to give us warning of any serious risk. Complacency would be foolish, especially as regards any increased firing of atomic bombs, but pessimism would be equally unreasonable.

Table 7.1 summarises the present situation. Radiotherapy is not listed separately; its contribution is almost insignificant. It involves large individual doses to a few, but this is of very minor importance to the population as a whole and in any case the patients are nearly all beyond reproductive age.

Table 7.1 Radiation to whole population

| Source of radiation | Dose as % of natural background |
|---|---|
| Natural background | 100% |
| Diagnostic radiology | 14.1% |
| Occupational exposure (medical, industrial, atomic energy) | 0.5% |
| Fall-out from nuclear explosions | 3.7% |

# 8. Cancer in Specific Sites – 1

*Everything's got a moral if you can find it.*
Lewis Carroll (Alice in Wonderland)

In this and the following chapters we shall discuss lesions which are treated freqeuntly, but by no means exclusively, in radiotherapy departments, or which show special features relevant to our subject. No attempt will be made to duplicate the standard textbooks of surgery. Instead a basic minimum of medicine, surgery, gynaecology etc. will be assumed. Our focus is on cancer in general and radiotherapy in particular. Hormones and cytotoxic drugs will be referred to where appropriate and then discussed in more detail in Chapters 12 and 13.

## Cancer of the breast

This is the commonest cancer in women (Table 1.2, p. 8). Only 1 per cent of breast cancer occurs in men and, next to lung cancer, it is the most common malignancy of all. Not surprisingly therefore, it forms an appreciable part of the work of a radiotherapy department, both in out--patients and on the wards. It illustrates well most of the principles and problems of cancer and its treatment.

The breast is an organ subject to repeated cyclical growth changes under the influence of hormonal stimulation, and the cells of the breast ducts, after repeated waxing nd waning of growth stimuli, are more liable than most cells of the body to take on irregular growth.

A 'lump in the breast' is by no means necessarily malignant. It might be a simple cyst, a patch of 'chronic mastitits', or fat necrosis. But every lump – or bleeding nipple – must be examined immediately and if the diagnosis is in doubt the mass should be excised for biopsy.

The treatment of breast cancer involves surgery, radiation, hormones and cytotoxic drugs. Let us say at the outset that the whole subject is one of complexity and uncertainty. Advancing knowledge has brought both enlightenment and improvement, but has also complicated the picture to such an extent that no two institutions – or even individuals – have quite the same policy of treatment, and here methods are more liable to change than with most other cancers.

*Natural history.* This is very variable indeed and depends on the inherent growth rate of the malignant cells. As for most cancers, there is a variable but relatively long pre-clinical period of development (see p. 21) but breast cancer is unfortunately more liable to throw off early secondaries, which remain silent for many months or long years. After diagnosis, some cancers run their full clinical course to a fatal end in a year or so, while others seem to enlarge only a little in the course of several years.

Even if no treatment whatever is given, the average length of survival is nearly three years, almost 1 in 5 (18 per cent) survive five years, while 1 in 25 (4 per cent) live for 10 years (Fig. 8.1).

In breast cancer therefore, the conventional five-year survival figure has very limited value. Ten-year figures are better, fifteen-year figures better still, but even after this interval, it is not completely safe to consider a patient 'cured' since recurrences and metastasis can still occur 25 years or more after initial treatment. It is still a controversial point, but after 15 years, in some cases at least, the expectation of life tends to be the same as that of the population as a whole, and in this sense it may be reasonable to regard cases as 'cured'.

*Staging.* Clinical staging is the most useful guide. Unlike cancer of the cervix, there is no widely accepted classification but the following is often adopted:

*Stage 1.* Tumour limited to breast tissue proper. No palpable nodes in axilla or elsewhere.

*Stage 2.* As in Stage 1, with axillary nodes palpable but mobile.

*Stage 3.* Local spread more advanced – skin nodules, peau d'orange, cancer-en-cuirasse, fixation to muscle or chest wall.

Nodes – axillary nodes fixed; may be palpable nodes above clavicle or in opposite axilla.

*Stage 4.* Distant spread has occurred – metastases in bone, lung, liver, brain etc.

*Lymphatic spread.* Figure 8.2 shows the principal routes – chiefly to axillary and internal mammary (parasternal) nodes, and thence to supraclavicular nodes.

*Blood spread* may be early or late-common sites of metastasis are bone, liver, lung and brain.

In the routine preliminary assessment of a case, in addition to clinical examination, it is usual to take X-ray films of the chest and skeleton (spine, ribs, pelvis) and clinically silent secondaries may (very infrequently) be discovered in this way. We also have more refined methods of detecting early secondaries. These include:

a. *mammography* of the other apparently normal breast;

b. *isotope bone scan* (see p. 52) which is able to show up secondary deposits in bone 18 months before they become large enough to produce radiological evidence on a film.

If secondaries are detected, the case becomes Stage 4. The newer techniques are expensive and time-consuming, and available in few departments as yet, but eventually they will be widely used. In fact, the day will come when scintiscanning will be used to detect occult secon-

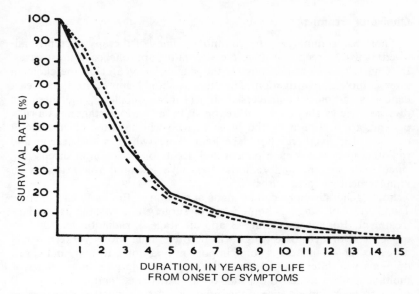

Fig. 8.1 Survival in untreated breast cancer. Data from three large series.

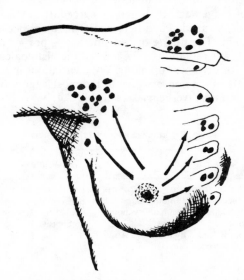

Fig. 8.2 Lymphatic drainage of the breast, showing axillary, parasternal (internal mammary) and supraclavicular lymph-nodes. Arrows show chief routes of spread.

daries in lung, liver and brain as well, in patients with apparently early breast cancer.

## Choice of treatment

Table 8.1 summarises the commonest lines of therapy currently advised. It will be seen that there are alternative approaches in most cases. In general treatment depends on the staging arrived at by the clinician after complete investigation. The student should appreciate that breast cancer is the most controversial subject in all oncology, and there are divergent views about optimal treatment in the various stages. As a rule, patients are first seen by the surgeon, who will have the chief voice in decision. Ideally there should be joint clinics where both surgeon and radiotherapist assess each patient and decide on policy after discussion, since both surgery and radiotherapy have essential roles to play in management of most cases.

Some generalisations can be made at the outset. For early cases (Stage 1 and most of Stage 2) some form of surgery is advisable as primary treatment. For most of Stage 3 and all Stage 4, radiation and/or hormones and/or cytotoxic drugs will be preferable. Most workers would agree so far — but it begs some important questions. In marginal cases, opinions will differ about 'operability', e.g. for a large primary mass or multiple axillary nodes. It depends on the experience (and temperament!) of the surgeon and likewise of the radiotherapist. Competent, experienced and honest doctors can arrive at different conclusions — for it is, in the end, a matter of judgement. If surgery is agreed, the extent of the operation has to be determined — and here again there are decidedly different schools of thought. The timing of radiotherapy — pre- or post-operative, and the necessity for radiation in the light of the histological findings, are further matters for divergent opinions. Wide variations in belief and practice exist from the most conservative to the most aggressive — hence the (perhaps bewildering) divergencies of Table 8.1.

Table 8.1 Management of breast cancer

|  | Aggressive | Conservative |
|---|---|---|
| Stages 1-2 | Radical mastectomy and Post-op. RT, especially if tumour anaplastic or in medial half or axillary nodes positive. Pre-op. RT used by minority. Adjuvant cytotoxics on trial. (Stage 2) | Local excision or simple (or extended simple) mastectomy and Post-op. RT (routinely or as in 'aggressive') |
| Stages 3-4 | RT to primary and/or painful secondaries. Simple mastectomy (early or late — e.g. 'toilet'). Post-op. RT ($\pm$ pre-op RT). Hormones as initial treatment, or for residues, etc. Cytotoxic drugs. | |

RT = Radiotherapy

It is reasonably certain that *in most cases the ultimate result is already predetermined at the time of diagnosis,* and depends on the biological nature of the individual growth, whether aggressive (with a short doubling time and high probability of early metastasis) or slow (long doubling time and late metastasis). This would account for the lack of improvement in mortality figures in the past half century, but still leaves room for heated argument of policy in particular groups or the individual case.

*The role of surgery*

Apart from rapidly growing anaplastic tumours, breast cancers are only moderately radiosensitive (less than squamous carcinoma) and as a rule cannot be reliably destroyed even by the largest tolerable doses of radiation. It is widely agreed, then, that for 'operable' cases surgery is the more reliable method of eradicating local disease. How extensive should the surgical procedure be? There are several possibilities:

1. Local excision of the tumour. (The monstrous word 'lumpectomy' has been coined – a barbarism which cannot be too strongly condemned).

2. Simple (local) mastectomy – removal of breast alone without disturbing the axilla.

3. Extended simple mastectomy – easily accessible nodes in lower axilla are also removed, but pectoral muscles left intact.

4. Radical mastectomy – pectoral muscles removed to expose whole axilla which is cleared of nodes as thoroughly as possible.

5. Super-radical (extended radical) mastectomy – the radical operation is extended to include internal mammary and supraclavicular nodes.

*Pros and cons of surgery.* Prior to 1950 the standard procedure was radical mastectomy. This was based on sound logical principles of cancer surgery, to remove the primary and regional nodes in one block of tissue. The extended radical carries the good logic even farther, but obviously increased morbidity (post-operative debility) and occasional mortality, and has never been widely practised. The chief drawbacks of radical operations are:

1. The cosmetic results in chest wall and shoulder regions are unsightly (evening dress and bathing suits are unwearable) and therefore psychologically undesirable. Nevertheless a low price to pay for cure.

2. Post-operative oedema of the arm is common – usually not very troublesome, but sometimes an appreciable handicap. Again generally acceptable in the interests of cure.

The radical operation is still widely practised (especially in U.S.A.) but recent years have seen a strong reaction against it, in favour of more conservative operations, especially simple mastectomy. There are several arguments in favour of simple mastectomy:

1. The psychological advantages of less mutilation and better cosmetic appearance.

2. Very much lower risk of oedema of the arm.

3. If there actually are no axillary secondaries, the radical is unnecessary. If there are involved nodes, modern radiotherapy is now known to be capable of eliminating them. The best results after radical operation are in those cases shown (by microscopic examination) to be free of axillary secondaries i.e. where the radical proved to be superfluous.

4. The long-term results of radical operations are not definitely superior.

This last point is of course the most important of all. Long years of experience and analysis of results, even after campaigns for earlier diagnosis and treatment, yielded a bitter harvest – the ultimate mortality rate obstinately refused to improve. The number of breast cancer deaths is as high now as ever.

Why does radical surgery so often fail, even in Stage 1 cases? The reason is to be found in the natural history of the disease and the liability to early metastasis, beyond the reach of any form of local treatment. This danger is even greater if there are secondary deposits in regional nodes, *for where regional nodes are involved, distant spread will already have occurred in most cases*. This accounts for the sharp decrease in survival when axillary secondaries are found:

## Five-year survival

Axillary nodes uninvolved     70 per cent
Axillary nodes involved       30 per cent

This means that the cases where growth is genuinely confined to breast and axilla only, are relatively few.

Disappointment in the long-term results of radical mastectomy led to a reappraisal. The best results of radical surgery were those cases with no axillary secondaries – i.e. cases where the radical procedure actually proved to be unnecessary. When axillary secondaries were present, radical operations were far less successful, and trial was therefore made of *less radical operations combined with radiation of regional nodes*. Follow-up results showed that 10-year survival rates were at least as good – Fig. 8.3. Hence the diminishing popularity of radical mastectomy in favour of more limited operations, especially simple (or extended simple) mastectomy. This has the advantage of a more acceptable cosmetic result, with the aid of a prosthetic artificial breast, and almost entirely avoids the risk of oedema of the arm. The combination of *simple mastectomy plus post-operative radiation* is now a line of management which is frequently followed, although many surgeons still practise radical mastectomy.

Distant spread may be clinically silent for years. But if it has occurred, then any form of local treatment, however drastic and extensive, is merely 'shutting the stable door after the horse has bolted'. Here then is our dilemma – how do we know in any given case, whether disease is truly

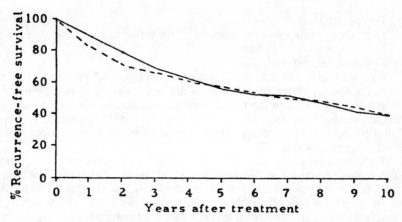

Fig. 8.3 Survival in breast cancer. Comparison of simple mastectomy with post-operative radiation (continuous line) and extended radical mastectomy (dotted line).

localised or has already spread beyond regional nodes? If it is localised, then radical local treatment could be life-saving. But in practice the number of such cases is low. Is then the policy of treating the many for the benefit of the few still justifiable? It is a genuine dilemma and there is room for differences of opinion. Hence it is not surprising that it forms one of the major controversies currently exercising the minds of surgeons and radiotherapists.

Some surgeons passionately contend that statistics are all very well in their place, but of no practical value for the individual surgeon faced with the individual patient. How can he be sure that radical operation would not save *this particular patient*? If so, would it not be unethical to deny her the possible marginal advantage, even if statistically insignificant? – a patient after all, is more than a statistic! At this point the argument tends to become philosophical and emotional rather than scientific.

The new techniques of detecting early and silent secondaries (see above) will help us to be more selective and save a proportion of patients from unnecessary and futile procedures. But our experience of these is very limited and the harvest has yet to come.

*Local excision* of the breast tumour alone is obviously attractive to the patient for its cosmetic and psychological advantages. Unfortunately it is unsafe, since we know from experience that microscopic foci of early malignancy are often present in the remainder of the breast in addition to the obvious clinical mass. However, the local procedure has its advocates on occasion, e.g. when wider operations are refused. With good fortune, perhaps with the help of post-operative radiation, it can at times succeed.

*The role of radiation in early cases. Stages 1 and 2*

In the early case, radiation is normally no rival to surgery, as we have seen.

The possibilities are:
1. Radical radiation – as substitute for surgery.
2. Pre-operative radiation
3. Post-operative radiation.

As shown in Table 5.1, p. 81, breast cancer belongs to the moderately sensitive group, where complete local disappearance is possible but not usual. Most growths in the breast itself are not good subjects for radical radiation, since we know from experience that viable residues are often left after full tolerance dosage. Hence surgery has usually no serious rival in the operable case.

Radiosensitivity varies with the degree of differentiation, and anaplastic growths can disappear rapidly under radiation. For this reason, if a growth is known to be histologically undifferentiated (Grade 3) or is growing rapidly with a short clinical history – which signifies anaplasia – primary radiation is preferable to primary surgery, especially if the growth is in the inner half of the breast or axillary nodes are palpable.

*The chief role of radiation is supplementary to surgery, usually following it.* Experience shows that mastectomy alone is followed by *local recurrence* in or near the scar in about 10 per cent of cases. Often the situation in the *regional nodes* cannot be known with any certainty from clinical examination – especially as axillary nodes can be felt in a third of normal women. If *axillary nodes* are palpably enlarged and considered clincially to contain secondary deposits, this will usually be confirmed on histological examination, but prove to be non-malignant hypertrophy in 20 per cent. If no significant axillary nodes are felt, subsequent histology reveals microscopic secondaries in at least 30 per cent.

*Internal mammary nodes*, lying deep to the chest wall, cannot be examined clinically unless grossly enlarged, but we know that they are invaded in almost a third of operable cases, in two-thirds when the primary is in the medial part of the breast, and in three-quarters when axillary nodes are invaded. *Supraclavicular node* enlargement is usually secondary to axillary or internal mammary invasion.

The object of *post-operative radiation* is to destroy any residual cancer cells in the chest wall or regional nodes, and so keep this whole area free of growth if possible. This is a worthwhile objective, since the presence of local disease, e.g. cancer-en-cuirasse on the chest wall – is liable to cause more suffering, especially mental suffering, than most distant metastases. The radiation fields generally include the skin flaps on the chest wall and all the regional lymph node areas – axillary, supraclavicular and parasternal – of the same side.

Radiation can begin as soon as the wound has healed, 10-14 days after operation. But if there is any doubt about the vitality of the skin flaps – infection, gaping of part of the wound, subcutaneous fluid – radiation should be postponed or abandoned. If the wound required a skin graft for closure, radiation should not be applied to it, as the blood supply on which its vitality depends is very vulnerable and necrosis and sloughing of the graft might easily follow.

*Pre-operative radiation* is less commonly used than post-operative. Its object is to destroy the more undifferentiated parts of the growth, which are likely to be at the edges – i.e. those cells which are most liable to give rise to recurrence and metastasis – and so reduce the risk of residual cells being able to 'take' in the skin flaps. Occasionally, both pre-operative and post-operative radiation is used.

In many centres, the combination of mastectomy (radical or simple, but especially simple) followed by radical radiation has become almost routine, particularly when axillary nodes are proved to be invaded. Figure 8.3 is good evidence of the value of post-operative radiation. However, a retreat from routine radiation is now evident, comparable to the retreat from radical surgery. In fact it is clearly evident after radical mastectomy and beginning to appear after simple mastectomy. Just as hard experience has shown that radical operations often do more harm than good and do not seem to improve the chances of survival, so we are now realising that the same may apply to routine radiation.

Another aspect that nowadays exercises our thinking is the *immunological* aspect. The defensive role of lymphoid tissue against invasion by cancer cells (see p. 15) is reason for caution in disturbing nodes not obviously invaded, and it seems at least possible that radiation can sometimes worsen the prognosis by damaging defence mechanisms.

To summarise, the problem of management of the early case is evidently very difficult and nurses must expect to find different regimes in different institutions. Some form of surgery is nearly always applicable, but there agreement ends. Clinical trials now in progress are expected to resolve some of the uncertainties in the next decade.

## Late Cases – Stages 3 and 4

These are defined on p. 112. Treatment here is essentially *palliative* and surgery usually contraindicated. In fact if it is used at the outset it will probably do more harm than good, as surgery involves cutting through lymphatic and other tissue containing cancer cells and, by the inevitable manipulation and squeezing of tissue, helps to promote both local and distant spread. If surgery is contemplated, pre-operative radiation is a useful precaution.

If the mass is bulky, or if the breast is of the big fatty pendulous type, which tolerates radiation poorly, local mastectomy should be considered with pre or post-operative radiation. This will be a matter of surgical judgment.

*Radiation* is generally the safest means of local treatment and the response may be very gratifying with long-term local control. If the response is not satisfactory, local mastectomy or excision may be worthwhile at a later date, if only for 'toilet' purposes, e.g. to remove a fungating mass.

In late cases, when surgery and radiation are no longer helpful, palliative treatment is continued, by *hormones* and/or *cytotoxic drugs*.

The overall picture of breast cancer, as it presents itself in clinical practice, varies with the type of patient (social class, education etc.) and is also influenced by health education, propaganda for early diagnosis and so on. But in this country and many others, we can make the following rough generalisations:

1. In any 100 consecutive unselected patients, 30 are inoperable when first seen.

2. Of the 70 operated on, only 35 are apparently free of disease after five years.

3. Of all the 100 cases therefore, at least two-thirds (30 + 35 = 65) are either inoperable or not cured by surgery in the limited sense of five-year freedom.

It follows that the role of surgery in treatment is inevitably restricted, while the role of other agencies, radiation, hormones and cytotoxic drugs is increasing.

*Adjuvant cytotoxic therapy* is an important recent innovation – see page 232.

### Radiation treatment and reactions

In the typical mastectomy case, post-operative radiation may be started as soon as wound healing is assured, even before discharge from hospital. Most or all of the course, which generally lasts 3-4 weeks, may be given on an out-patient basis. These patients, who are relatively fit, are therefore not usually seen on radiotherapy wards.

Treatment is conventionally daily, Monday to Friday; but sometimes on alternate days, Monday, Wednesday, Friday. Until recently, orthovoltage (deep X-rays – see p. 00) was widely used, but megavoltage (including cobalt beam) is now replacing it in many centres. Treatment is directed to the whole of the chest wall, to include the skin flaps and all the regional lymph node areas (Figs 8.4, 8.5). There may be separate fields for axillary-supraclavicular and parasternal regions, while the chest wall is treated by tangential fields instead of direct fields, to minimise dosage to lung tissue. Nurses should see actual marking-up of fields in the treatment department and setting-up on the treatment couch.

The treated area is necessarily large and the total dose is about 4000-4500 rads, depending on the voltage and overall time. Since breast cancer is only moderately radiosensitive, dosage has to be taken to tolerance levels, and skin reactions – mild, moderate or severe – are to be expected. The earliest and most marked occurs in the axilla, due to moisture and friction. Skin reactions usually reach their height about a week after the end of treatment. There will be at least dry desquamation and usually some patches of moist desquamation (see p. 88-9).

Treatment of skin reactions is along the lines laid down on p. 90-2, and in most cases healing is rapid and uneventful in 2-3 weeks. If there is an

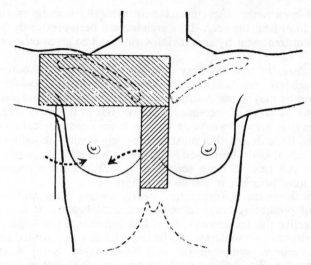

Fig. 8.4 Technique of X-ray treatmrent in breast cancer. Four fields are shown – 1. Axillary-supraclavicular. 2. Parasternal. 3 and 4. Chest wall tangential (the breast may or may not be present). A posterior axillary field is usually added. (*Jones, in Robinson's Surgery, Longmans*)

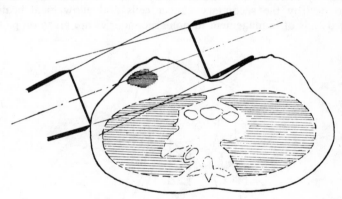

Fig. 8.5 The two tangential fields of Fig. 8.4. This technique spares the normal lung tissue.

unexpectedly severe reaction due to idiosyncracy, admission to hospital and treatment as for burns may be indicated, but this is rarely required.

## Palliative treatment for recurrences and metastases

These are common and any radiotherapy ward is likely to have several cases.

*Local recurrence* after mastectomy typically occurs as small skin nodules in or near the scar. If the area has not been previously irradiated, out-patient treatment by superficial X-rays can be given over one or two weeks.

*Metastases in bone* are very common and a frequent source of pain, e.g. 'lumbago' or 'sciatica' from deposits in lumbo-sacral spine. Radiographs may show destructive changes as areas of rarefaction, occasionally as areas of increased sclerosis, but in the early stages symptoms may be present weeks or months before radiological changes are apparent. Bone destruction must be relatively great — actually two-thirds of a vertebral body destroyed — before radiological diagnosis becomes possible. An isotope bone scan (see p. 52) will often demonstrate a deposit long before it is visible on a film.

X-ray treatment is, fortunately, nearly always successful in relieving pain and promoting bone sclerosis and local healing. It is remarkable how effective this treatment can be. For instance, a whole pelvis riddled with destructive secondaries can be healed and reconstituted so that the patient becomes symptom-free and walks again. X-ray fields of appropriate size (Fig. 8.6) are used, giving, e.g. 2000 rads in five sessions.

*Pathological fracture* may occur in a long bone, e.g. femur or humerus. The orthopaedic department may be called on to stabilise the fragments by inserting an intramedullary pin. Radiation may then be given to destroy the secondary cancer cells and allow local healing. Further details of management in bone secondaries are given on p. 169.

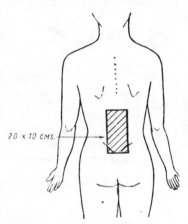

20 × 10 CMS.

Fig. 8.6 X-ray field to lumbar spine, to treat secondary deposits from breast cancer.

*Cerebral metastases* may cause various neurological symptoms including personality changes. Their presence can sometimes be demonstrated by an isotope brain scan (see p. 52). Radiation of the brain by megavoltage (3000 rads in 10 sessions) may give excellent palliation.

*Effusions* may occur in pleural or peritoneal cavities due to secondary deposits. If they recur after tapping, they can usually be prevented from rapidly reaccumulating by injection into the cavity of a cytotoxic drug such as mustine (see p. 221) or a radioactive isotope such as gold, yttrium or phosphorous (see pp. 201-2).

*Other metastases* may occur in almost any organ, especially lungs and liver. Occasionally local radiation may be worthwhile if the patient's general condition is good enough, but at this stage of dissemination hormones and cytotoxics are more likely to be used.

### Breast cancer and pregnancy

After treatment, younger patients are often advised to avoid further pregnancy. However, after a year's freedom from recurrence or metastasis, this policy is not necessary. In fact, the evidence goes to show that subsequent pregnancy, if anything, does more good than harm, especially in those under 35.

Breast cancer discovered during pregnancy can present difficult problems. The interests of both mother and child must be considered, and they may at times conflict. Tumours tend to be more anaplastic in pregnancy and the prognosis rather worse than average, but by no means hopeless.

The normal principles apply as far as possible.

In the first-half of pregnancy, mastectomy (radical or simple) should be performed. On post-operative radiation opinions differ. The risk to the mother from residual malignancy has to be balanced against the risk to the child from scattered radiation. At this early stage of development the child's tissues are extremely vulnerable even to low doses of radiation. On the whole, radiation is better avoided; if there is residual malignancy, the prognosis for the mother is poor in any case.

In the second half of pregnancy, if the growth seems early and not enlarging aggressively, it may be left and treated after the delivery. If growth is rapid or in Stage 3, the interests of the mother should prevail – pregnancy should be terminated and the lesion treated. If the child is viable, Caesarian section should be performed, followed by mastectomy.

Breast cancer appearing in lactation is apt to grow rapidly. Lactation should be suppressed (by drugs) and treatment carried out on the usual lines.

### Cancer of the uterine cervix

Cancer of the uterus is one of the commonest cancers in women (see Table 1.2, p. 8) and the second commonest female cancer in radiotherapy departments. Growths of the cervix (Latin for 'neck') outnumber those of the corpus (Latin for 'body'), though the incidence of the latter is increasing.

Radiation treatment of cervical cancer is one of the greatest triumphs of radiotherapy. It has been developed over many years and is now so well established that it plays a dominant role in management.

*Staging* (Fig. 8.7). There is an internationally accepted classification as follows:

*Stage 0* Carcinoma-in-situ, also called pre-invasive carcinoma or intra-epithelial carcinoma.

*Stage 1* Growth confined to cervix or spread upwards to involve corpus.

*Stage 2* Growth has spread beyond cervix; either to vaginal fornices, or to parametrium, but not as far as lateral pelvic wall.

*Stage 3* Spread has extended as far as lateral wall(s) of pelvis or has reached the lower third of vagina.

*Stage 4* Growth has involved mucosa of bladder or rectum or has spread outside the true pelvis.

*Carcinoma-in-situ* is a most important lesion, as it is often the precursor of invasive cancer and can be detected by *cervical smears* in 'well' women. Its place in screening programmes and early cancer detection has been described on pp. 35-6.

*Lymphatic spread* is to nodes alongside the uterus, then into the various pelvic groups (iliac, hypogastric, obturator, sacral), and from these upwards to paraortic nodes. Late spread to inguinal nodes can occur via the round ligament or from the vulva, but it is rare.

Clinical staging, as always, is not a good indication of the true (i.e. pathological) extent of spread. A seemingly early Stage 1 lesion with a small primary on the cervix, may have microscopic but impalpable secondaries in pelvic nodes. We know, in fact, that there are actually involved nodes in about 20 per cent of Stage 1 cases, and far more frequently in later stages.

Lymphography is a recent addition to pre-treatment assessment. If invasion is detected, this must be taken into account in the plan of treatment (see p. 176).

*Treatment – Surgery or radiotherapy?*

For late cases – Stages 3 and 4, which are in any event inoperable – there is no question that radiation is the method of choice (just as in late breast cancers). For early cases – Stage 1 and many of Stage 2 – surgery and radiation are alternatives. Before the days of radium treatment, the only hope of cure lay in *radical hysterectomy,* i.e. removal of the uterus with a generous vaginal cuff, tubes, ovaries and as much pelvic soft tissue as practicable, including all regional lymph-nodes if possible (Wertheim's hysterectomy). The picture has now changed completely and most cases are treated by radiation. This is not to say that surgery has no place in treatment or that there is no room for divergent opinions – far from it!

*Stage 0.* This is still a puzzling situation, reflecting our lack of precise knowledge of the natural history of cervical cancer. The optimal management is still doubtful and controversial. Follow-up studies have shown that while many cases proceed to invasive cancer, many others do not,

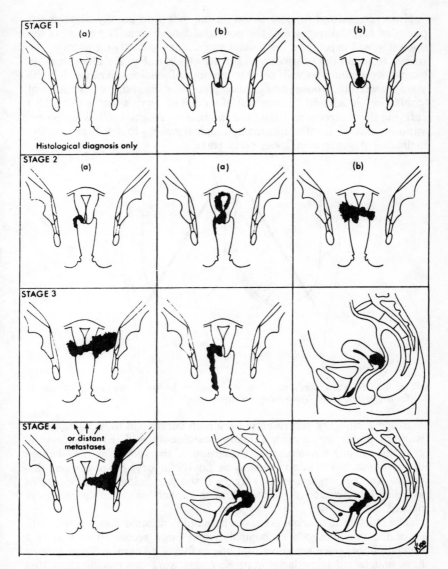

Fig. 8.7 Illustrations of the stages of cancer of the cervix. For details see text. (*Jeffcoate,* '*Principles of Gynaecology*', *Butterworths*)

and the suspicious changes regress spontaneously. It may therefore sometimes be justifiable to wait and rely on close follow-up observation to see whether the appearances persist or improve.

However, natural anxiety to be on the safe side usually dictates the policy of surgical removal of the potential danger area. The extent of the operation will depend on the patient's age, and especially on whether she wishes to retain the possibility of further children. For the older woman, simple hysterectomy will be the method of choice; likewise for the younger woman, whose family is complete. For the rest, the operation of 'conisation' is advised i.e. removal of a cone of cervical tissue (Fig. 8.8.) carrying the danger area round the external os. Regular follow-up observation is essential, with repeated cytological smears to detect any further malignant degeneration at an early stage.

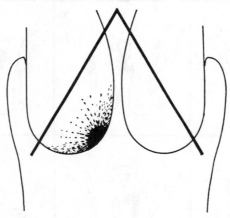

Fig. 8.8. To show the area of cervix removed by the operation of conisation. *(Jeffcoate, Principles of Gynaecology, Butterworths)*

*Stage 1.* Surgery and radiation are both curative in most cases. Some workers prefer surgery for (a) adenocarcinoma and (b) endo-cervical growths causing barrel-shaped expansion of the cervix, as they believe the response to radiation tends to be unsatisfactory; other workers disagree. Another argument for surgery is the psychological advantage of avoiding all reference to radiation and its implications in an apprehensive patient.

The chief controversial point — where opinions still differ — is the ability of the two methods to control lymph node secondaries. This is a crucial factor, since we know that one in five of all clinical Stage 1 cases have undetected secondaries in pelvic nodes. Surgeons usually claim that surgery is more reliable here, but we now have proof that radiation is also capable of eliminating pelvic node metastases.

The statistical test of experience is the best available. On the basis of long years of observed results, most gynaecologists are satisfied that on balance, with average surgical skill and average radiotherapeutic resources, the results of radiation are superior to those of surgery — and this is the simple reason why most cases are now managed by radiotherapy alone. In this respect the situation differs widely from breast cancer.

The mortality from radiotherapy is almost nil, and the morbidity very low. Surgical mortality and morbidity have declined over the years, but are not negligible. The dangers of, e.g. damage to ureters and urinary fistulas are still harrowing surgical possibilities. Some workers have tried to get the best of both worlds by giving full radiation followed by radical surgery; this is excellent in theory, but carries the possible complications of both. If surgery is used as principal treatment, a single pre-operative radium insertion to moderate dosage is advisable; this gives good protection to the vaginal vault against local recurrence.

Occasionally, a radiation failure, which can occur even in Stage 1, can still be rescued by operation.

*Stage 2.* There is less controversy than for stage 1, though still a place for surgery in cases with minimal extension beyond the cervix, especially for the exceptions noted under Stage 1. The standard treatment is intracavitary radium (usually two insertions) followed by external megavoltage.

*Stage 3.* Radiation is almost the only treatment possible. One intracavitary insertion (or two) may be followed by external radiation, alternatively external radiation alone. Good palliation is usually achieved, and a proportion of lasting results. Some of the latter may be due to the fact that palpable parametrial induration may be more of inflammatory than malignant nature – clinical examination cannot distinguish.

The scope of surgery is restricted to heroic efforts necessitating removal of bladder and/or rectum also (with diversion of bowel and/or ureter) – called 'pelvic exenteration', e.g. in a desperate attempt to salvage a radiation failure. Morbidity and mortality are inevitably high

*Stage 4.* Palliation is the aim here, and clinical judgment may suggest that it is kinder to withhold radiation, and keep the patient as comfortable as possible by nursing care and sedative drugs, especially in the elderly. Radiation can be useful, e.g. in controlling bleeding and discharge or pain. Attempts at intracavitary treatment are liable to precipitate fistulas, by rapid local destruction of growth precariously plugging bladder or rectum, if not by mechanical trauma.

Surgical exenteration can be considered if the patient is fit enough.

Table 8.2 lists the usual methods of treatment for the various stages.

### Contra-indications to intracavitary treatment

In addition to those already mentioned the following situations make surgery preferable:

a. Pelvic infection, e.g. salpingitis, past or present. Radiation may light up a seemingly quiescent infection.

b. Pelvic adhesions from old or recent infection or surgery in the pelvis. A loop of bowel readily becomes adherent to pelvic structures

Table 8.2 Treatment of carcinoma of cervix

| | Usual treatment | Exceptional treatment | Point | Dosage (rads) Radium | MXR | Ra + MXR |
|---|---|---|---|---|---|---|
| Stage 0 | Conisation or Hysterectomy | Observation | | | | |
| Stage 1 | Radium with or without MXR | Hysterectomy | A | 6000 | 1500 | 7500 |
| | | | B | 1500 2 insertions | 3500 | 5000 |
| Stage 2 | Radium plus MXR | Hysterectomy | A | 6000 | 1500 | 7500 |
| | | | B | 1500 2 insertions | 3500 | 5000 |
| Stage 3 | Ra. plus MXR or MXR alone | Exenteration | A | 4000 | 3000 | 7000 |
| | | | B | 1000 1 insertion | 4000 | 5000 |
| Stage 4 | No specific treatment or MXR | Exenteration | Treatment according to case. Usually MXR. Pelvis up to 5000. | | | |

Overall treatment time − $4\frac{1}{2}$ to 5 weeks.

(uterus, etc.). The bowel's normal mobility gives it considerable protection from radiation damage − to which it is much more vulnerable than uterus or bladder. An adherent or trapped loop of bowel can receive damaging dosage especially from an adjacent intracavitary source, with resultant ulceration, haemorrhage, diarrhoea, even perforation, and later fibrotic constriction and obstruction.

c. Uterine fibroids (benign fibroblastic tumours of uterine wall) may distort the cavity and make insertion difficult. Radium may also cause acute necrosis in the fibroid, leading to a surgical emergency.

*Radiation technique*

The patient is admitted to hospital a day or two before operation, to allow time for routine investigations (blood count, blood urea, I.V.P. etc.) and transfusion if necessary. Full preparation for operation is carried out.

In the theatre the lithotomy position is usually adopted, though some therapists prefer the knee-chest position, which makes it easier to pack the vaginal applicators away from the rectum. After careful inspection and manual examination of vagina and pelvis to determine the full extent of the growth, cystoscopy is usually carried out, to inspect the base of the bladder for evidence of malignant invasion. A self-retaining catheter is then inserted.

The basic principle is the *intra-cavitary insertion of radioactive sources* in uterus and vagina. Actual techniques − types of applicators, radium content and period of insertion − differ from one centre to another, but the fundamental principles are always the same.

The uterine canal is gradually dilated until it will accommodate an intra-uterine tube about 6 cm long and 0.8 cm wide. When the operator is ready for actual insertion, the nurse brings the tube, and attached nylon cord, from behind its protective lead barrier in the corner of the theatre, and with the aid of long-handled forceps, hands it to the operaor who inserts it as rapidly as possible. Then, with similar precautions, the vaginal applicators (one or more sources) are inserted up against the cervix at the vaginal vault. Their cords extend outside the vagina along with that of the uterine tube and are attached to the thigh by adhesive strapping. Where appropriate, the procedure is completed by plugging the vagina with a gauze pack, beginning behind the vaginal applicators so as to increase their distance from the rectum and prevent them slipping out of position.

In the theatre it is important to observe all the protection precautions described on pp. 101-105.

After the operation, the patient is wheeled on a trolley to the X-ray diagnostic department and films are taken of the pelvis – antero-posterior and lateral. Better still, films are taken in the theatre itself, with a mobile diagnostic set. These are inspected to ensure that the radium sources are lying in proper position. If the operator is dissatisfied, e.g. the intra-uterine tube may have slipped down so that it is lying partially or wholly in the vagina – the patient may have to be brought back to the theatre and the applicators re-inserted; or, if she is on the ward, they may be removed without delay.

There is no 'standard' technique, not only because different centres use methods which differ in detail, but because treatment must be individualised to suit the individual patient. The chief cause of difficulty lies in the variable state of affairs found at the vaginal vault. For example, the vaginal part of the cervix may have disappeared, eroded by the growth, or a bulky growth may make it difficult to position the vaginal sources satisfactorily, or the fornices may be so contracted that there is simply not enough room at the vault for the applicator. Therefore treatment must be tailored to fit the patient and applicators of different sizes must be available so that the most suitable can be chosen.

*Applicators.* The intra-uterine tube is fairly standard and contains about 50 mg of radium. Figures 8.9, 8.10 and 8.14 show it in position. Vaginal applicators contain a total of about 60-70 mg and are rather variable in design – three types are illustrated in the figures. Those in Fig. 8.9 are oval in shape, and two of these 'ovoids' are placed side by side in the fornices as shown. They are made of hard rubber or plastic and the radium tubes occupy the centre of the long axis.

The applicators of Figs. 8.10 and 8.11 are made of plastic and are kidney-shaped. One or two are mounted by sliding on a long central metal tube and cylindrical segments are then added, to fill the rest of the vaginal length. The external vertical end-piece completes the whole applicator and is secured by straps to a belt fastened round the patient's waist, so that the whole applicator is firmly fixed and cannot rotate. The

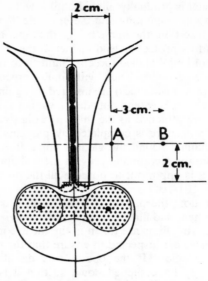

Fig. 8.9 Diagrammatic uterus and vagina, showing intra-uterine tube, cross-sections of ovoids in lateral fornices, separated by spacer, and points A and B. (*Paterson, Treatment of Malignant Disease, Arnold*)

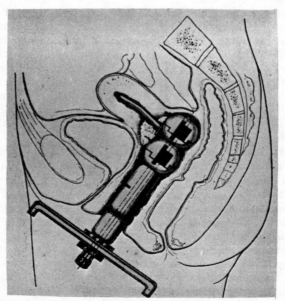

Fig. 8.10 The Sheffield applicator in position, with two radium-holding 'kidneys' and uterine tube.

radium tubes are inserted – inside or outside the theatre, behind lead plates – into the selected size of box-like 'kidney' (Fig. 8.11) and small heavy metal inserts of tungsten are placed behind the tubes. These absorb about half the gamma rays in the posterior direction and so give considerable protection to the patient by reducing the dose to the rectum. With this technique there is no need to plug the vagina with a gauze pack, which is somewhat irritant and may promote infection.

The radium remains in the patient for about two days. For Stages 1 and 2 a second insertion is made a week or 10 days later. In another technique, only a single insertion is made, which remains in for five days continuously – though the packing and applicators may be removed at intervals for cleaning and re-insertion.

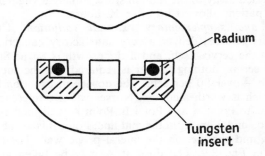

Fig. 8.11 Cross-section of kidney-shaped vaginal radium holder, showing position of radium tubes and removable tungsten inserts. If tungsten protection is not required, plastic inserts are used instead. The radium tubes are then inserted on each side and the applicator closed by the cap.

*Caesium 137* has largely replaced radium, because of its various advantages (see p. 56). But no new principles are involved.

*On the ward,* precautions must be observed, as described on p. 103. The patient is not allowed out of bed for toilet or other purposes. Most therapists insert a catheter into the bladder at the time of radium insertion, and the bladder is emptied into a bag at the bedside. Some prefer the patient to pass urine naturally, to reduce the risk of bladder infection, but this involves more exposure for the nurse (bedpans etc.) and is undesirable. Full use should always be made of mobile lead screens if available, to protect the nurse at the bedside.

Slight pyrexia is usual following radium insertions, but a four-hourly record must be kept and evidence of infection reported. Latent pelvic infection may have been exacerbated, or the fundus of the uterus may have been perforated during operative procedures, with resultant peritonitis. If so, it may sometimes be necessary to remove the radium prematurely.

The patient is nursed flat on her back, which is very tedious for her, but avoids dislodging applicators. Leg movements and deep breathing exercises should be carried out. Pressure areas, especially in the scapular region, should be powdered twice daily and bed sheets straightened but not changed unless soiled.

Vulval pads need regular inspection and changing if soiled. If there is any suspicion of misplacement of radium holders, the doctor must be informed at once.

All nursing procedures should be as expeditious as possible, and all nurses and other ward staff should minimise the time spent near any patient carrying radium sources. The necessity for this should be explained to the patient, so that she will not feel neglected.

When the time comes for removal of the radium the pack (if any) is removed first, then the vaginal containers withdrawn by their cords, then the intra-uterine holder. They are placed at once in the lead box which is then wheeled away to the radium store. Finally a vaginal douche is given and the patient allowed up after 12 hours.

*Dosage and supplementary external radiation.* Utero-vaginal intracavitary sources deliver a very satisfactory cancericidal dose in the region of the cervix itself, and if the growth is a true Stage 1, involving only the cervix, nothing further is required and the success rate will be very high — over 90 per cent. The dosage distribution is shown in Fig. 8.12, which is worth studying. Nurses will see references on treatment sheets etc. to Point A and Point B. Point A is defined as 2 cm above the external os and 2 cm from the mid-line; Point B is at the same level but 5 cm from mid-line, i.e. on the lateral pelvic wall. These points are also marked in Fig. 8.9. The dose at A may be taken as critical for the primary growth, while that at B is relevant for regional lymph-nodes. Hence dosages are commonly assessed in these terms.

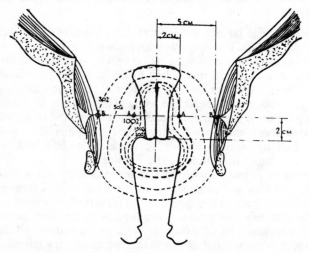

Fig. 8.12 Isodose curves in the pelvis for a typical radium distribution. The position of points A and B is shown. (*Tod, British Practice in Radiotherapy, Butterworths*)

We can never be sure from clinical examination alone whether metastases are present in pelvic nodes. Even in Stage 1 cases one in five will have early secondaries there. Radium cannot deliver a cancericidal dose much beyond Point A and any involved nodes near B will be underdosed. Most workers, therefore, supplement intra-cavitary treatment with external radiation – megavoltage X-rays or cobalt beam – to bring the dose at Poont B up to a suitable level for all cases, with the possible exception of the smallest Stage 1 lesions.

This supplement is commonly given after the second radium insertion, over a period of about three weeks. In more advanced cases, especially Stage 3, only one radium insertion is given and the rest of the treatment (the major part) carried out by external radiation. The same may be done for Stage 4 cases, but here many prefer to rely entirely on external treatment.

The external radiation may be given partly before and partly after radium insertions or between two insertions. The usual type of field is shown in Fig. 8.13. The central strip is 'blacked out' by a thick metal filter in the middle of the beam, which absorbs most of the radiation in the middle of the field. This is to protect the midline structures, especially bladder and rectum, as well as the cervix itself which receives adequate dosage from the radium, and to concentrate the dosage on the outer parts of the parametria and pelvic walls, increasing the dose near Point B. If radium is not used, i.e. in advanced cases, the central strip filter is of course unnecessary.

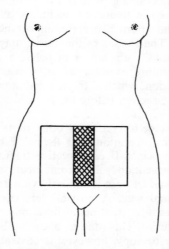

Fig. 8.13. X-ray or cobalt-beam field for supplementary radiation to pelvis. The central strip filter cuts out most of the radiation to mid-line structures (cervix, rectum, bladder). A similar field is applied at the back.

In this way the intra-cavitary and external radiation are dovetailed to give the dosage required, and care must always be taken that safe tolerance levels are not exceeded. The radiotherapist will have charts available in the theatre to give him at least an approximate idea of the doses at important points – at A, B, bladder and rectum. In awkward cases the physicist will be called in, to work out doses more accurately with the help of the X-ray films taken after the insertion. These figures will be available in the radiotherapy department so that the megavoltage doses at A, B etc. can be fitted in, to give the final combined doses required (Table 8.2).

If paraortic nodes are also treated, the fields will resemble Fig. 9.8, p. 164. The dose to the paraortic section should not exceed 4500 rads.

*Early radiation reactions.* The cervix and body of uterus are unusually tolerant of high dosage. The more vulnerable organs that are potential sources of trouble are – rectum, bladder and any loops of bowel trapped or adherent in the pelvis. As we have noted, special precautions are taken routinely for rectal protection – packing or heavy metal filter. A minor degree of rectal irritation with perhaps slight diarrhoea, is usual after a radium insertion, and settles rapidly. During external radiation symptoms may reappear and be quite troublesome. Treatment may then have to be slowed down or suspended for a few days.

Bladder irritation, with dysuria and frequency, is another possibility, but less common. Skin reactions are unlikely to give trouble if megavoltage is used.

*Late reactions and complications*

a. *Infection.* An ulcerated growth is always more or less infected. The manipulations involved in treatment, including dilatation of the uterine canal, may spread infection; hence the importance of full surgical antiseptic precautions. The fundus of the uterus may be perforated by the exploring uterine sound, with danger of pelvic and peritoneal infection. The patient's temperature is observed after insertion; an unusual rise points to pelvic infection, which is treated with antibiotics. It may be advisable to remove the radium before the prescribed time rather than risk spreading infection.

b. *Bowel.* Overdosage to rectum or other parts of the bowel can lead to late haemorrhage, ulceration and fistala. Fibrotic narrowing and obstruction can also occur. If conservative treatment does not lead to healing, surgical intervention will become necessary.

c. *Bladder.* The bladder base is similarly vulnerable, lying just in front of the anterior vaginal wall. A possible late reaction is telangiectasia months or even years after treatment; these may bleed and cause blood in the urine (haematuria). This may be alarming but is rarely dangerous and soon settles. Cystoscopy, however, is advisable, to exclude a more serious cause of bleeding. *Vesico-vaginal fistula* (communication direct from bladder to vagina with constant leakage of urine) is almost always due to advanced growth rather than radiation damage.

With modern technique, these complications are becoming rarer, and one must remember that radical surgery has an equally formidable list of unpleasant complications, such as injury to the bladder, ureters or rectum, ischaemic necrosis of the ureter (because of impairment of its blood supply) leading to fistula, ureteric incompetence, and stress incontinence of the bladder.

*Terminal illness*. In failed cases, death is usually due to local effects in the pelvis, from ureteric obstruction leading to renal failure and uraemia. This is in contrast to breast cancer, where the end comes from metastatic growth in distant organs.

## Cancer of the cervical stump

Subtotal hysterectomy, i.e. removal of the uterus above the level of the cervix (e.g. for fibroids) was commonly practised in former times, but now given up. Carcinoma may develop in the remaining stump. Radium treatment is difficult, as the length of canal left is rarely enough to hold a radium tube. Vaginal applications can be made, supplemented – or replaced entirely – by external radiation.

## Results of Treatment

Over the years, results have steadily improved, owing to better technique, concentration of treatment in skilled hands at large centres, and earlier diagnosis and treatment. Twenty-five years ago, the overall five-year survival rate was 30 per cent, now it is 50 per cent.

In Stage 1 cases, radiotherapy alone gives a five-year survival of 70 per cent and at the best clinics the figure is 85-90 per cent. The comparable five-year figure for Wertheim's hysterectomy in Stage 1 is 65 per cent and in the hands of a few very experienced surgeons 80-90 per cent.

Experience with combined radium and surgery is not yet extensive, but the results bid fair to be an improvement on either alone – especially in Stage 2 cases.

The conclusion is clear – with average facilities and skill, radiotherapy offers the best chance in most cases.

The survival rates in advanced stages are of course poorer – falling to 0.5 per cent in Stage 4.

*Cancer of the cervix in pregnancy*

About 1 per cent of cases are discovered in pregnancy and the prognosis is less favourable, because the hormonal and vascular changes predispose to rapid growth and spread, while the pregnancy itself is a hindrance to treatment.

Abdominal hysterectomy and Wertheim's hysterectomy, with various combinations of radium etc. have been used, but the modern trend favours full radiation in most cases, regardless of the pregnancy.

In the first six months, with the fetus non-viable, external megavoltage should be used, giving 1000 rads to the pelvis weekly for four weeks. The fetus will be killed and after two or three weeks abortion will usually occur. At the end of the course, the uterus will be sufficiently involuted for treatment to be continued by intra-cavitary radium to usual dose levels. If abortion does not occur, hysterectomy should be performed.

In the last three months, with a viable fetus, Caesarean delivery should be performed, followed after a few days by external radiation and completed by intra-cavitary radium as above. Some prefer to apply intra-vaginal radium first, regardless of radiation effects on the fetus, which usually survives. This is followed by Caesarean delivery or hysterectomy. It is never advisable to induce abortion before giving radiation, as this gives the worst results of all.

Occasionally, in the sixth month or so, a decision may have to be taken whether or not to wait a short time for viability, in the hope of a live child. This is an ethical problem of balancing the interests of mother against child. The wishes of the family should be taken into account after full discussion and explanation.

With skilled treatment, five-year survival figures are 40-50 per cent.

## Cancer of the uterine body

The epithelial lining of the uterus is the endometrium (Greek 'endo' = within, 'metra' = womb). Endometrial cancers are becoming more frequent. The typical age is 50-60, higher than for cervical cancer but 25 per cent of cases occur before the menopause. It has no relation to parity and is as common in nuns as other women — quite unlike cervical growths.

The standard treatment is surgical — *total hysterectomy* — in early operable cases where there are no contraindications such as hypertension, diabetes, obesity etc. Inoperable cases, e.g. appreciable extension outside the uterus, or cases technically operable but unsuitable for surgery, are treated by radiation — either intra-cavitary radium, external radiation or a combination of the two.

Even for operable cases, results are definitely improved by combining surgery with radiation. This decreases the risk of local recurrence at the vaginal vault, which is a serious hazard of surgery alone. The best combination is *pre-operative utero-vaginal radium,* usually a single insertion, and surgery can follow in a week or two — or up to six weeks later. Others prefer *post-operative radium,* with applicators inserted at the vaginal vault to deal with any residual cells in the suture area.

If radiation alone is used, *intra-cavitary radium* insertion is carried out on similar lines to the technique for cervical cancer. Figures 8.14 and 8.15 show two examples. Two insertions are usual and if there is evidence of spread beyond the uterus, supplementary external radiation to the pelvis should be added, as in Fig. 8.13.

*Results.* This lesion is one of the more curable cancers. For operable, i.e. early growths, the overall five-year survival rates are 60-70 per cent after hysterectomy. For patients under 60, it can be as high as 85 per cent.

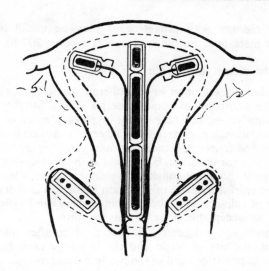

Fig. 8.14 A radium technique for body of uterus. Similar to treatment of cervix, but with two additional small containers inserted first at the upper end. Note the flat boxes, each holding four small radium tubes, inserted in the lateral fornices. (*Marie Curie Hospital*)

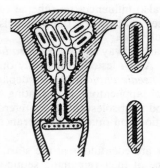

Fig. 8.15 Two types of Heyman applicators, and a uterine cavity packed with as many as it will hold. Note the flat box of radium against the cervix, and the eyelets in the applicators for threads. (*Hulbert, in 'Treatment of Cancer in Clinical Practice', Livingstone*)

Radiotherapy is not often used alone, unless surgery is contraindicated or the lesion too advanced, but can achieve figures of 45-60 per cent. At one centre, which has specialised in treating endometrial cancers by radium alone, survivals over 80 per cent have been achieved – Fig. 8.15 shows the technique developed there.

*Metastases* may occur at any time and one of the commonest sites is the vagina. If surgical excision is impracticable, good results can be obtained by local radium – either intra-vaginal or needle implant.

*Hormone therapy* with progestogens may be useful in advanced, recurrent or metastatic endometrial cancer (see p. 207-8).

## Cancer of the mouth and throat

This is relatively common in radiotherapy wards, because radiation is usually the treatment of choice (see pp. 83-4). Surgery is an alternative in many cases, but necessarily involves a more or less serious degree of mutilation, e.g. glossectomy, whereas radiation can restore normal anatomy and function. If radiation fails, surgery may still be possible later. But if bone (or cartilage) is involved at the outset – e.g. mandible – primary surgery should be considered, since radiation is less likely to be curative. The chief drawback of radiation is the residual dryness, owing to inhibition of salivary and mucous glands. This can be distressing, but is generally an acceptable price to pay for cure.

In addition to age and general condition, which often rule out surgery in any event, the site of origin and the histology must be considered. Some sites, e.g. posterior third of tongue, tonsil and nasopharynx, are unsuitable for surgery, not only because of the mutilation involved, but because the growth is commonly a poorly differentiated histological type (anaplastic) which tends to throw off early metastases, but is responsive to radiation. Finally, the presence or absence of palpable secondary nodes in the neck will also influence the scheme of treatment. Clearly, joint consultation between surgeon and radiotherapist is important for individual decision in each case.

Treatment is now nearly always by *external radiation* – megavoltage X-rays or cobalt beam. A few lesions, especially on the tongue, are still best treated by *radium needle implant*. A few departments still use *surface radium* on special applicators for treating lip, hard palate or alveolus, but this method is obsolescent. Here reference should be made to pp. 92-3 where reactions on mucous membranes and their treatment are described.

*Teeth.* Many patients are edentulous at the start, others obviously require complete clearance of their remaining septic stumps, but in some cases – especially in younger patients – it may be difficult to decide whether to advise prophylactic removal of healthy teeth. The problem is discussed on p. 93. If need be, the patient should be reassured that dentures can and will be fitted later after the mouth has healed – but this may be many weeks or months, when tissue shrinkage is complete.

With an ulcerated carcinoma, some degree of infection is inevitable and food residues may add to the debris. *Mouth toilet* is an important part of the whole regime of treatment and full use should be made of frequent mouth washes especially after meals. Any bland antiseptic will do, though none is better than plain sodium bicarbonate – a teaspoon to a pint of warm water.

*Radium needle implant*

This used to be the commonest method of treating cancers in the mouth (tongue, floor of mouth, buccal cheek, faucial pillar), but is now used mainly for early lesions of the anterior two-thirds of the tongue. We shall describe such a case. Expert nursing plays an important part.

It is good practice to explain to the patient in advance what is going to be done and that he need not fear pain, but should expect some discomfort and dysphagia.

Radium needles are described on pp. 54-5. The radiotherapist works out in advance, from the dimensions of the lesion, exactly what needles he will require, i.e. the appropriate length and radium content. These are removed from the radium safe, threaded with strong silk knotted close to the eye of the needle) with the help of a lead block (Fig. 7.4, p. 103) on a protected bench. Sterilisation is either by heat or chemical methods (e.g. ethylene oxide). Safety precautions in the theatre – lead L-plates, long-handled forceps, speed and distance – are comparable with those in intra-cavitary gynaecological work. The assisting nurse hands each needle to the operator as required, after grasping it by the long-handled introducer (Fig. 8.16) and lifting it from the lead block.

General anaesthesia should be intra-tracheal. The jaws are separated by a gag, the tongue is grasped with tongue forceps near the tip, and a small pack is inserted into the pharnyx to catch blood trickling from the mouth. The operator inserts the needles one by one in the predetermined pattern, so that the implant covers the whole growth with a safety margin of at least 1 cm. Each needle is pushed home, so that its eye is covered, just beneath the mucosal surface, by pushers (Fig. 8.16) and the silk is then stitched to the tongue with a suture (No. 2 chromicised catgut and a small round-bodied fully curved needle). When all the needles have been inserted, the silks are counted and gathered together outside the mouth and strapped to the cheek, so that if a needle works loose it will not be swallowed. To avoid possible trauma by rubbing on the angle of the mouth, they may be passed first through a soft rubber tube. The pharyngeal pack is removed and blood etc. aspirated from the pharynx.

On return from the theatre, constant supervision is necessary until full consciousness is regained, in case of respiratory difficulty or attempts by the semi-conscious patient to pull the needles out.

Immediately after the operation, if possible, radiographs are taken, to check the lie of the needles. If any serious errors of positioning are seen, it may be necessary to bring the patient back to the theatre for correction of the implant. The films also assist the therapist and physicist in working out the dosage and time with accuracy. A typical distribution is shown in Fig. 8.17. An average length of time for the implant is about seven days giving a dose of about 6000 rads.

The patient should be allowed up next day, which is good for both morale and hygiene and lessens the risk of chest complications, but he must not be allowed to leave the ward alone. The needles should be

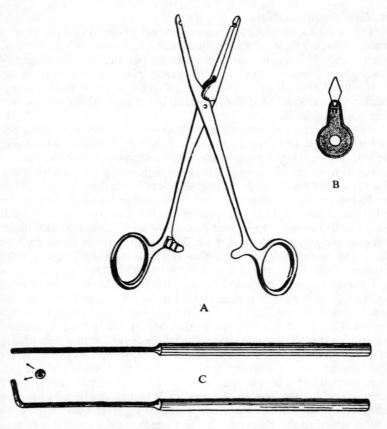

Fig. 8.16 Instruments used in radium needle implant work. A, Needle introducer – note the grooves near the end, to grip the needle. B, Needle threader. C, Pushers, straight and angled, to complete the insertion of needles. (*Paterson, Treatment of Malignant Disease, Arnold*)

checked daily, by counting the number of threads; if any are missing, or if a needle appears misplaced (e.g. if the head is showing), the doctor should be informed at once.

Mouth toilet is important, but swabs should not be used while needles are in, as they are painful and may even dislodge needles or sutures. Four-hourly irrigations should be carried out, and gentle syringing or spraying may be helpful.

Nutrition is important. Drinking is liable to be difficult because of local discomfort and oedema. A feeding cup with soft rubber tubing on the spout is helpful, or else simple straws. Fluid intake should be watched and fruit drinks with extra glucose given. Patients may need considerable encouragement and coaxing to maintain adequate fluid and nutrition.

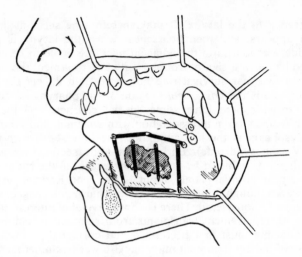

Fig. 8.17 Diagram of radium needles for single-plane implant in the tongue. (*Paterson*)

Needles are removed at the appointed time (see p. 104). No anaesthesia is required and there is seldom any real difficulty. It is usually carried out by the doctor, but can be done by an experienced nurse. The sutures are cut if necessary and the needles usually slip out easily with a slight pull. One or two of them may require a little instrumental leverage of the needle head before they can be extracted without pain. The patient is then given a hot drink and a sedative. The needles must be counted and returned to the radium store with the usual precautions.

The radiation reaction of mucositis usually sets in within a few days of removal, with membrane formation as described on p. 92. This should not be mistaken for thrush, but if there is any doubt a swab may be taken. Full healing with disappearance of tumour and re-epithelisation of ulcerated surfaces, should be complete in 3-6 weeks, depending on the size of the lesion.

Instead of radium (or cobalt or caesium) needles, gold grains (pp. 56 and 202) can be used as *permanent implants*. These are useful particularly for old people, as they allow free tongue movement and so lessen the risk of complications. Iridium wire is another possibility (p. 204) especially for the posterior part of the tongue.

*Results* in lesions of moderate extent that can be adequately covered by needling, as in Fig. 8.17, are usually excellent in experienced hands.

### External radiation

Most lesions of mouth, pharynx, nose and sinuses, are now treated by megavoltage or cobalt beam.

In the hypopharynx, the commonest growth involves the *pyriform* (or piriform – Latin for 'pear-shaped') fossa, the small cul-de-sac at the side of the entrance to the larynx. It may therefore be silent at first, until dysphagia appears, and then hoarseness when the larynx is invaded. Lymph-node secondaries in the adjacent neck are liable to be early and may indeed be the first sign of trouble. With any treatment the outlook is poor, with a five-year survival rate not more than 25 per cent.

A nearby site is the *post-cricoid* region at the pharyngo-oesophageal junction. Growths here have some special characters – they occur typically in women, often in association with anaemia, and gradually increasing dysphagia is the key symptom (the Paterson-Brown-Kelly or Plummer-Vinson syndrome). Early lymph-node secondaries are common. Treatment is liable to be unrewarding except in the earliest stages, and the five-year survival is only about 10 per cent. Radical surgery is a possibility, even though it involves extensive pharyngolaryngectomy, and should always be considered. There is now a revival of interest in surgical attempts, with replacement transplants from stomach or colon. In any case, the anaemia must first be treated and corrected.

A course of radical treatment may take 3-6 weeks. Sometimes the first part of the course at least can be taken as an out-patient, but it is advisable to be in hospital during the height of the reaction, i.e. towards the end of the course and following it.

The general picture and management of skin and mucosal reactions have been outlined on pp. 88-93. With megavoltage, skin reactions are hardly ever a problem and rarely proceed to more than a little dry peeling. But mucosal reactions can be severe, prolonged and a great strain on the patient, depending on the size of the irradiated fields, especially if through-and-through treatment, using bilateral fields, is given to mouth or pharynx.

Careful attention is needed to diet – protein concentrates, feeding cups and straws, avoidance of irritants like pickles or vinegar. Fluid intake is very important, as dehydration can be insidious; if there is any doubt, a fluid balance chart should be kept. Dryness of mouth and throat, with viscid and diminished saliva and mucus, will need frequent mouth washes. Dysphagia may be helped by aspirin mucilage or benzocaine lozenges before meals.

Reactions may persist for many weeks and even cause trouble for months. The strain should never be under-estimated and, in addition to expert nursing on the ward, a period of prolonged convalescence is often indicated.

*Split course therapy*

Many patients will be elderly and have extensive disease when first seen. Even here, some degree of regression is usually obtainable, sometimes surprisingly good, and useful palliation can be achieved with great improvement in comfort. For these patients the aim should be to *avoid severe radiation reactions* completely, giving cautious treatment, e.g. 1000 rads weekly for two weeks, then two or three weeks' rest, then another fortnight's treatment, another interval of rest, then another fortnight's treatment, as indicated by clinical progress.

Split courses of this kind call for considerable experience and judgement on the part of the radiotherapist. They have their inconveniences, both for the patient and treatment staff, but can be very rewarding and should be used more frequently than they are.

## Maxillary antrum

Carcinoma arises from the internal lining of the cavity, but clinical signs are usually due to extension through the antral walls – to nose, ethmoids, cheek, mouth or orbit. *Radiation is the treatment of choice,* in spite of bone invasion, but drainage of the cavity should first be established, e.g. by palatal antrostomy. Careful field planning with megavoltage beams is carried out, and in order to cover the full spread of growth with a safe margin it may be necessary to include the ethmoid cells and the whole orbit, with no attempt to spare the eye, since this would risk missing part of the growth. Radiation conjunctivitis will follow, and is treated as described on p. 95.

After full radiation, some workers explore the antrum surgically and remove suspect patches. Late cataract will be inevitable and possibly retinal degeneration with loss of vision.

The five-year survival is about 25 per cent, and higher for early cases.

## Nasopharynx

Surgical removal of growths is rarely practicable, but radiation can give good results. Patients may present with local symptoms (blockage of Eustachian tube and deafness, or nasal blockage), but very often the first evidence of cancer is from secondary nodes in the upper neck, maybe bilateral. Invasion of the base of the skull is also common, with cranial nerve palsies; or of the orbit, with proptosis.

Histologically most are either anaplastic, including the so-called lympho-epithelioma because of the association of lymphocytes, or lymphosarcoma, and it may be very difficult for the pathologist to decide whether it is anaplastic carcinoma or reticulosis. The anaplasia accounts for their tendency to early node metastasis in the neck.

Treatment of this type of growth should include the whole of the neck, from base of skull to clavicles, whether nodes are palpable or not, because of the high probability of microscopic secondaries. Their radiosensitivity is high enough to enable a cancericidal dose to be given to this large block of tissue – 4000 rads in four weeks. This will produce a severe mucosal reaction, but this is justified as cures can be obtained even in unpromising cases.

## Cancer of the larynx

This may arise on the vocal cord (glottic – the commonest type) or below the cord (subglottic) or above the cord (supraglottic). The classical early symptom is hoarseness and early diagnosis is therefore possible.

The vocal cord itself has very few lympathic vessels and as long as the growth is still confined to the cord, lymph-node metastases in the neck are very unlikely. But once it has transgressed the cord, the rich lymphatic supply causes a much higher incidence of secondaries.

Treatment of glottic lesions, especially with the cord(s) still mobile, is one of the triumphs of radiotherapy, and the success rate in early cases is 85-90 per cent at least. Surgical excision by *laryngofissure* (splitting the larynx in the midline and retracting the two halves laterally to permit removal of the growth) is equally successful, but always leaves an impaired voice. Radiotherapy on the other hand ensures a normal or near--normal voice and is thus clearly superior. Even if the cord is fixed, radiation should still be used, for though the prospects of cure are not so good, a failure may still be rescued by surgery (laryngectomy).

*Radiation technique* is simple, but must be meticulous. It employs megavoltage, preferably on an in-patient basis, though out-patient treatment in favourable circumstances is not ruled out. Either a parallel pair or a wedge pair of fields is adequate (Fig. 5.4, p. 77) with a dosage of 6000 rads in five weeks. The post-radiation reaction of mucositis with accompanying soreness, dryness, dysphagia etc. will follow the usual course, and should settle down within a few weeks.

*For more advanced lesions,* especially with perichondritis of the laryngeal cartilages, surgery is probably the treatment of choice, since control by radiation is very unlikely and the presence of persistent oedema and infection makes life a misery. If surgery (laryngectomy) is unacceptable, cautious radiation should be tried.

*Tracheostomy* is sometimes necessary for obstruction of the airway by an advanced growth and this will complicate the radiation technique. It will not be practicable to make a shell for beam direction (see p. 78) but with megavoltage, radical radiation is still feasible, and it is often possible to close the tracheostomy later.

### Lymph-node metastases in the neck

In many cancers of head and neck, the prognosis depends more on the presence or absence of secondaries in cervical nodes than on the primary growth.

As a generalisation, it may be said that *operable nodes in squamous carcinoma are best treated by surgery,* usually radical block dissection. Some workers now advocate external radiation (megavoltage) and claim equally good results. Inoperable nodes must rely on radiation as a second best.

However if the primary is anaplastic – e.g. many growths of the posterior third of the tongue, the faucial and naso-pharyngeal regions, surgery is likely to be ineffective and radiation is preferable, especially as secondary nodes are liable to be bilateral. In many of these cases the lesion is sufficiently radiosensitive to allow the whole of the neck as well as the primary to be treated in one block to a cancericidal level of dosage – see under 'Nasopharynx' above.

Radiation is also indicated in preference to surgery in all cases of reticulosis, e.g. lymphosarcoma, using large fields to include the whole of the neck.

## Cancer of the oesophagus

This constitutes about 5 per cent of all cancers and is one of the most serious of all, as cure by any means is rare. The leading symptom is dysphagia, first for solids and finally for fluids. Investigation includes a *barium swallow,* when the limits and length of the growth should be assessed, especially the lower end. *Oesophagoscopy* should provide confirmation by biopsy. Growths are squamous carcinoma, except at the lower end where adenocarcinoma is found, best regarded as cancer of the stomach with spread to the oesophagus.

Even though local cure is sometimes obtainable, the outlook is poor because even in small growths – 5 cm long or less – 50 per cent have secondary nodes in the neck, mediastinum or upper abdomen, while in larger growths the incidence is 90 per cent.

Treeatment is either by surgery or radiation and every case is a matter for joint consultation. If the patient is in good condition, and there is no evidence of extensive local fixation or secondaries, resection is advisable – especially for adenocarcinomatous growths at the lower end, which are radio-resistant and require *gastro-oesophagectomy.*

Many patients are in anything but good condition, with loss of weight, even emaciation, anaemia and dehydration. The most rapid relief in such cases will come from passing a Ryle's tube, if possible, at the time of oesophagoscopy, after which nutrition can be restored and further treatment considered.

*Radical radiation* is a practicable alternative to surgery, but only if the general condition is good and the growth is estimated to be not longer than 5 cm, otherwise the treated volume will be too large to tolerate curative dosage and in any case success will almost certainly be nullified by secondaries. If there is doubt on these points, radical radiation should not be attempted, since the whole course and post-radiation reactions are a considerable strain even on a fit patient.

If it is decided to irradiate, very careful tumour localisation and beam direction are essential, and the technical problems are a great challenge to the radiotherapist (see pp. 74-9). The treatment scheme must be worked out in the planning department and care must be taken to minimise dosage to spinal cord and lung tissue (see p. 76). A typical three-field megavoltage scheme is shown in Fig. 5.3, p. 77. The dose aimed at is 5000 rads in four weeks with fields of about 15 × 5 cm.

The radiation mucositis will cause considerable soreness and add to the dysphagia temporarily. No specific treatment for this is available, but nursing care on the lines laid down on pp. 92-3 is indicated, but is better may become necessary in some cases for severe reactions, but is better avoided since it carries some danger of perforation of the oesophageal wall, with resultant mediastinitis that is virtually untreatable.

At megavoltage, skin reactions will be negligible and present no nursing problems, but convalescence is bound to be prolonged. In a successful case, dysphagia will be relieved when reactions have settled in a few weeks, and progress can be observed at follow-up fluoroscopy.

*Palliative treatment.* In practice it is usually only a minority of cases that can be considered suitable for radical treatment of any kind and a decision must then be made as to the best mode of palliation. Apart from purposive inactivity plus morphia — the kindest way for the very advanced case — the alternatives are:

1. Palliative radiation.  2. Intubation.  3. Gastrostomy.

*Palliative radiation* to a lower dosage than a radical course may provide some relief for a few months at most, but the price in discomfort for the patient is high — probably too high for the short-lived benefit, if any.

*Intubation* is the palliative method of choice. Tubes of the Souttar type are now out of date and in any case tend to be dislodged. A Mousseau-Barbin plastic or (better) a soft rubber Celestin tube with a flanged upper end should be used. A gastrotomy is necessary to enable the tube to be drawn down into the stomach, but it should ensure adequate swallowing for the rest of the patient's existence.

*Gastrostomy.* This is a theoretically attractive short-circuit to maintain nutrition, but its obvious drawbacks make it rarely advisable. If it is to be considered, the problem should be fully discussed with the patient's family, in the light of the prognosis and the very doubtful balance of pros and cons.

*Pre-operative* radiation prior to resection has some advocates now and may have something to add to the prognosis but the case remains to be proved.

The overall 5-year survival is about 5-10 per cent; for growths in the neck, 10-20 per cent. The lower third fares better, with about 30 per cent after surgery.

Some of the best results come from Japan, after an aggressive policy of pre-operative radiation plus surgery.

## Cancer of the gastro-intestinal tract

Growths of stomach and bowel, especially colon, are among the commonest cancers of all. With few exceptions — they are adenocarcinoma. In general, surgery is the treatment of choice. Cancericidal doses of radiation are not tolerated, and attempts at radical treatment lead to ulceration, perforation and obstruction. Damage to kidneys is another limiting factor.

*Malignant lymphoma* may occur, especially in the stomach and local node involvement is usual. Diagnosis is usually made on laparotomy or even only after gastrectomy has been performed. If removal appears complete and the nodes are free, no further treatment is necessary. Usually, however, additional therapy is indicated, to include the whole of the stomach (if still present) and regional nodes. External radiation is given with large fields (localised with the help of barium), which must of necessity include the left kidney and cross the midline to the right, but the right kidney must be avoided. A tumour dose of 3000-3500 rads is given in 4 weeks.

*Cancer of the rectum* is of interest to the radiotherapist especially since the advent of megavoltage. Surgery is still the first choice in operable cases, but local recurrence is common, causing pain in sacral and perineal areas, maybe radiating down lower limbs. For advanced inoperable or recurrent cases radiation can often give worthwhile palliation. Simple antero-posterior pelvic fields of about 14 × 12 cm are used, to give a depth dose of about 4500 rads in 4 weeks.

Small perineal recurrences may receive a direct field on cobalt beam, with applied bolus.

*Pre-operative radiation* of about 2000-3000 rads before the radical operation for removal of the rectum seems to be of real value in improving the long-term results. It is now under trial and if confirmed will be widely adopted as a routine.

### Cancer of the anus

Anal cancers are mostly of aquamous type and show the same kind of radiosensitivity as squamous carcinoma elsewhere. Growths of the anal canal are usually adenocarcinoma and similar to rectal growths. Small lesions may be successfully treated either by surgery or radiation. The best radiation technique is a needle implant. If is often desirable to perform a colostomy prior to radiation; this can be closed later if treatment is successful.

Larger growths, if unsuitable for surgery, can be treated by external radiation, using simple fields, wedge pairs or other appropriate techniques.

# 9. Cancer in Specific Sites – 2

*What I tell you three times is true.*
Lewis Carroll (The Hunting of the Snark)

## Lung cancer

Numerically, this is the most serious problem of all, and becoming rapidly worse (Table 1.2, p. 8). We have already discussed several aspects, under carcinogenesis (p. 13), epidemiology (p. 32), early detection (p. 34), prevention and education (pp. 38-43).

The *presenting symptoms* are typically cough, dyspnoea, haemoptysis or chest pain, from the primary lesion. But they may come from *secondaries,* long before the primary gives any trouble – e.g. bone pain or pathological fracture from a deposit in a long bone; neurological effects (epilepsy, palsies) from cerebral secondaries; enlarged supraclavicular nodes; skin nodules etc. There may be venous and lymphatic *obstruction* from enlarged mediastinal nodes, with oedema of neck, face and arms; *hoarseness* from involvement of the recurrent laryngeal nerve in the thorax; *dysphagia* from pressure on the oesophagus; enlarged liver etc.

Growths at the apex of the lung are liable to invade the brachial plexus and sympathetic nerves, producing severe pain in the shoulder region and arm (Pancoast tumour and syndrome).

In all cases a full assessment should be made, including bronchoscopy and biopsy if possible, to determine the extent of the primary and the presence or absence of metastases. On the basis of the findings, two vital decisions must be made:

1. Is it operable or inoperable?
2. Is treatment to be radical or palliative?

*Treatment* is by (1) surgery (2) radiation (3) cytotoxic drugs – or combinations of these. Hormones have no part to play.

1. Surgery – lobectomy or pneumonectomy – is the best hope of success, but the overall results are lamentable. Of all patients seen by the surgeon, a third are clearly inoperable at the outset, another third are found to be inoperable in the theatre at thoracotomy, while the remaining third are apparently resectable. Actually, the operability rate is only 10 per cent of all cases, and the five-year survival after pneumonectomy only 25 per cent. The sad fact is that at least 75 per cent of resected cases die with secondaries, which usually precede diagnosable disease. In sum, *less than 5 per cent are successfully treated by surgery.*

2. Radiation is the first alternative to surgery, and as usual there are two possibilities – (i) radical (ii) palliative treatment.

i. *Radical radiation* can be considered for a growth that appears truly localised and is not too large – e.g. if surgery is contraindicated or is refused. Careful planning and beam direction are necessary (pp. 74-9) and the scheme of treatment will resemble Fig. 5.3, p. 77, taking care to minimise dosage, as far as practicable, to spinal cord and normal lung tissue. The patient should be in hospital and the course may last 4-6 weeks, with a tumour dose of 4500-6000 rads.

It is not usually possible to avoid the oesophagus, and dysphagia is therefore a likely complication, beginning during the treatment and lasting for several weeks after the end. A late reaction is lung fibrosis; at high dosage, some degree is inevitable, and it can be serious and disabling.

Most lung cancers are moderately radiosensitive, and the anaplastic type (the 'oat cell' carcinoma – so called from the elongated appearance of the cells resembling oat grains) highly so, so that local cure is often obtainable. Surgeons have learnt from experience not to embark on surgical treatment of oat-cell carcinoma. Apart from this type the results of radiation in operable cases are inferior to those of surgery. In practice, radical radiation is not commonly attempted, and in some centres hardly ever, but an occasional success is attained.

ii. *Palliative radiation* is usually the best means of relief in the inoperable or advanced case, and in many centres is the treatment given at some stage to most patients. It is a very valuable agent and gives great, if temporary, benefit to large numbers for whom no other relief is readily available.

Its use is for *palliation of symptoms,* but if symptoms are not very troublesome, it is generally *wiser to withhold treatment* until they do become troublesome. This is paradoxical and contrary to sound general principles of early treatment. It is certainly tempting to push treatment at an early stage, as likely to achieve more benefit, but in practice it does not prolong life in the incurable case, and may preclude effective palliation later on when symptoms are serious. Moreover, the patient is liable to attribute his later deterioration to the previous radiation.

Relief is usually obtainable for cough, dyspnoea, haemoptysis and pain. A blocked bronchus may be re-opened, with drainage and relief of infection. Simple technique should be used – e.g. two fields, front and back, and the course may last about a week, with moderate dosage, e.g. 1750 rads. Out-patient treatment is usually satisfactory.

Good palliation is usually also achieved in *mediastinal obstruction. Bone secondaries* respond well as a rule, and a single treatment of 1500 rads may suffice for relief of pain.

*Paraplegia* may result from compression of the spinal cord by extradural deposits. Surgical decompression (laminectomy) is sometimes justifiable for this, and in any event the deposits should receive fractionated external radiation. See also p. 153.

*Cerebral secondaries* are commoner from lung cancer than from any other primary. They are treatable in the same way as those due to breast cancer (p. 122).

3. Cytotoxic drugs (see Chapter 13) are of definite value in some cases, especially for the anaplastic (oat-cell) type. The most frequently used drugs are mustine and cyclophosphamide. They can be combined with radiation – e.g. a short course of intravenous cyclophosphamide may be given first, then radiation, and maintenance drug therapy afterwards.

They have emergency value in mediastinal obstruction and early paraplegia, especially if radiation is not – or not immediately – available. They may also help in obstruction if radiation tolerance has been exhausted by previous treatment.

*Pleural effusion* is common, from involvement of pleural surfaces. External radiation rarely helps, but following removal of most of the fluid by paracentesis, a cytotoxic drug can be instilled into the pleural cavity (e.g. 20 mg of mustine). This may control effusion for weeks or months. An alternative method of intra-cavitary treatment for effusion is by a radioactive isotope (gold, yttrium or phosphorus – see Chapter 11).

*Conclusion.* Clearly, the treatment of lung cancer is a most unsatisfactory business. Surgery helps only a tiny minority, and radiation is only a temporary palliative for the many. Our best hope lies in prevention. It is not a flattering thought, but it is a sober fact that at least 90 per cent of lung cancer is now preventable ... if only ...!

## Secondary cancer in lung

This is very common indeed, but not often treatable by any method. As a rule, lung secondaries are multiple and herald the beginning of the end, with short life expectancy. But there are exceptions, and a patient may survive in good condition for several years after secondaries become visible on a chest film – e.g. in some salivary gland or thyroid cancers, and some slow-growing sarcomas. On rare occasions, a genuinely solitary secondary in the lung has been removed by lobectomy and the patient apparently cured – e.g. in carcinoma of the kidney.

In the vast majority of cases, neither surgery nor radiotherapy has anything to offer, though hormones or cytotoxic drugs may cause temporary improvement in appropriate cases of hormone dependence. If radiation is used, it will usually be in some form of chest 'bath', and to give useful results the tumour must be more radiosensitive than the surrounding normal lung tissue. Otherwise, effective doses would cause severe radiation pneumonitis, which would itself probably be fatal, if the patient survived long enough. However, there are a few instances where growths are so radiosensitive that adequate dosage can be given without excessive lung damage – some reticuloses, seminoma, dysgerminoma, chorionepithelioma, nephroblastoma (Wilms's tumour) and neuroblastoma. In these, radiation chest baths for secondaries can even be curative at times.

### Intracranial tumours

A list of the commonest of these is given in Table 2.2, p. 25. Their curious names stem mostly from Greek roots (see Appendix, p. 263). We shall not attempt to explore the subject deeply, for the field is rather specialised, a matter for the neurological surgeon and neuropathologist. Fortunately, they hardly ever metastasise outside the central nervous system (brain and spinal cord).

Half of all primary brain tumours are *gliomas,* and of the many varieties of non-glial tumours the commonest is the meningioma. But the commonest intracranial tumour of all is not included in the list – i.e. *secondary deposits* (single or multiple) from a primary growth elsewhere. In fact, 5-10 per cent of all cacners give rise to cerebral secondaries. The most frequent primary sources are lung and breast (not surprisingly, as these are the commonest cancers in males and females).

The *diagnosis* and *localisation* of these lesions may include special investigations – electro-encephalography, ultrasonic and radioactive brain scans, cerebral angiography and ventriculography – in addition to ordinary radiographs and lumbar puncture. The latest diagnostic aid, perhaps the most valuable of all is the computer – assisted tomography of the EMI scanner (EMI = Electronic & Musical Industries). The clinical syndromes cover a very wide general and neurological field – cranial nerve and other motor and sensory defects, hemiplegia, epileptiform fits, drowsiness and unconsciousness, headache and vomiting, mental and personality changes, loss of memory, incoherence of speech, irritability, restlessness or even violence, retention or incontinence of urine and faeces, etc. They present formidable problems on the ward, and tax all the resources, skill and patience of the nursing staff.

*Treatment.* The initial treatment of most primary tumours is nearly always surgical, but complete removal is only exceptionally possible. Post-operative radiation is therefore commonly added, in the hope of improving results. Its value in most cases is not great, but it can increase survival in some patients, especially the younger. With some exceptions results are poor, life expectancy short, and most treatment is essentially palliative.

Patients should be warned to expect loss of hair, though it may grow again in the course of months, depending on age and dosage. A wig can always be supplied for temporary or permanent use. Radiation treatment takes 3-4 weeks, and dosages must not exceed about 4000 rads, otherwise the vascular damage will lead to brain necrosis. Late brain damage is thus a possible danger, and the effects can easily be mistaken for recurrent growth.

*Medulloblastoma* is a tumour arising in the cerebellum of children, usually aged between two and seven. It spreads by surface routes via cerebrospinal fluid to the rest of the brain and spinal cord. Treatment begins with craniotomy for biopsy, partial removal and decompression, followed by radiotherapy. To cover the total possible extent of spread, the whole of the brain and spinal cord must be irradiated.

A long narrow posterior field covers the spine, widening at the top to include the head (Fig. 9.1). An anterior field to the head completes the scheme. Fortunately this tumour is very radiosensitive, and doses of 3500 rads in five weeks can be given safely. Long-term successes are obtainable in about 25 per cent of cases. Some impairment of bone growth is inevitable, but is not gross. Medulloblastoma is an example of lesions where *radiation has revolutionised the prognosis of* what was otherwise a hopeless cancer.

*Pituitary tumours* are a special and fascinating group. They include the chromophobe, eosinophil and basophil adenomas. Though they are technically simple tumours and never metastasise, they can be dangerous because of their size and produce *pressure symptoms,* especially on the neighbouring optic chiasma, with resultant visual field defects and partial or complete blindness (especially the chromophobe adenoma).

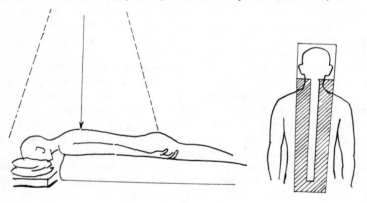

Fig. 9.1 Posterior field to include the whole cranio-spinal axis. The spinal part is demarcated by lead protection (cross-hatched).

In addition, the *hormonal disturbances* have far-reaching effects, including acromegaly (from eosinophil adenoma) and Cushing's syndrome (from basophil adenoma).

*Treatment* should be surgical if vision is threatened. Since complete removal of tumour is not possible, it is generally wise to add post--operative radiation to forestall recurrence. If vision is satisfactory, radiation is a good alternative to surgery and will usually relieve pressure symptoms, including headache. A four-week course of external radiation to 4000 rads is given, using narrow beams or rotation.

*Secondary deposits* in the brain are very common and give rise to hemiparesis, convulsions, headache, vomiting etc. They can often be localised by an isotope brain scan (p. 52). In rare instances they may be solitary, and surgical removal may even be possible. Usually this is impracticable, and external radiation may relieve symptoms, e.g. a fortnight's treatment by a simple parallel pair of lateral fields giving 3000 rads. Alternatively, oral dexamethasone (8 mg a day) may be used first, to control symptoms by lowering intracranial tension.

## Spinal cord compression

This is a serious condition, often insidious, leading to paraplegia and incontinence if not relieved. Diagnosis is often late, when neurological damage has become irreversible. Many growths can produce secondary deposits causing progressive compression – usually extradural, e.g. breast, lung, Hodgkin's disease.

To be effective, treatment must be early, at the stage of initial motor or sensory disturbances in the lower limbs or of bladder upset. These cases are emergencies, and the quickest and most effective treatment is surgical – i.e. decompression by laminectomy, if the patient's general condition permits, with partial removal of the offending mass.

In some cases, e.g. reticulosis, radiosensitivity may be high enough to justify preliminary treatment by radiation directed to the appropriate spinal level indicated by the neurological signs. If this does not lead to rapid improvement, laminectomy should be done. Cytotoxic drugs may also be useful in these emergencies, but local radiation is usually less upsetting and more reliable.

If caught and treated in time, compression is usually relieved, and the patient is spared the misery of terminal paraplegia and incontinence.

## Cancer of the bladder

This is one of the cancers which is now increasing in frequency, and the cause probably lies in the urinary excretion of carcinogenic irritants derived from the environment (see p. 13).

There is an exceptionally high incidence in some (sub) tropical countries notably Egypt, due to the frequency of *bilharziasis* involving the bladder. This is a water-borne parasitic infection carried by snails; the organisms penetrate the skin and eventually eggs are formed which have a characteristic terminal spine. These lodge in the bladder wall and cause intense inflammatory changes and ultimate malignancy.

Stones (calculi) in the bladder are not causative factors.

Neoplasms of the bladder range from benign papilloma to invasive carcinoma. *Papillomas* may be single or multiple, and are best treated by cystoscopic diathermy. But they are very liable to recur and give rise eventually, perhaps after repeated fulgurations, to invasive cancer. They should therefore be regarded as *pre-malignant* and kept under regular observation by periodic cystoscopy.

*Preliminary investigation* consists of:

1. Examination of urine – the centrifuged deposit may also be examined microscopically for malignant cells.

2. Blood chemistry – urea, electrolytes, etc.

3. Intravenous pyelography – to detect hydronephrosis from obstruction, assess renal function and exclude primary growths of kidney and renal pelvis, which can produce secondary seedlings in the bladder.

4. Cystoscopy under general anaesthesia, to include bimanual examination for assessment of depth of growth and extent of local invasion.

5. Biopsy via operating cystoscope.

Complete co-operation between urological surgeon and radiotherapist is vital in the management of bladder cancer. They should have a joint clinic and joint cystoscopy sessions in the theatre, so that the full extent of invasion and spread can be estimated and the optimum treatment decided for each case.

As usual, division into Stages is desirable (Fig. 9.2):

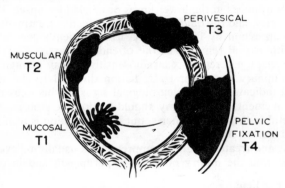

Fig. 9.2 Staging of bladder cancer. (*Wallace, Tumours of the Bladder, Livingstone*)

*Stage 1*. Limited to mucosa and submucosa.

*Stage 2*. Extending into, but not through, the muscular wall.

*Stage 3*. Extending through the bladder wall (extravesical or perivesical).

*Stage 4*. Fixed or fixing to neighbouring organs or pelvic wall; or lymph-node or other secondaries present.

## Treatment

Stage 1. For small superficial lesions, single or multiple, *closed endoscopic resection and diathermy* via the operating cystoscope is the method of choice. All visible lesions should be destroyed at one session if possible. It is a time-consuming procedure calling for considerable skill and patience. Stay in hospital is short, but cystoscopy should be repeated monthly until the bladder mucosa is clear, with further fulgurations if necessary.

The intervals between follow-up cystoscopies can then be lengthened to three months, then six months and finally a year – but the patient must not be discharged. Haematuria at any time, of course, calls for immediate cystoscopy. In this way, early growths can often be controlled for many years.

Open *diathermy* or *excision* by suprapubic cystotomy should only be done if endoscopic technique is not possible. It is particularly undesirable for frankly malignant growths, as there is a high risk of implanting cancer cells in the incisional lines of the bladder and abdominal wall.
Stage 2. The alternatives are:
1. Partial cystectomy.    2. Total cystectomy.    3. Radical radiation.
*Partial cystectomy* is possible for growths far enough away from the trigone, with re-implantation of the ureter if necessary. But the results are apt to be disappointing. *Total cystectomy* is theoretically sound, but involves urinary diversion, which is always a formidable matter and fraught with unpleasant consequences. The ureters may be:
a. Transplanted into the colon – i.e. uretero-colostomy – with considerable danger of overwhelming ascending infection and pyelonephritis, electrolyte disturbances, hydroureter and hydronephrosis.
b. Brought out on to the abdominal surface; a urinary bag must be worn, and the skin is liable to excoriation.
c. Implanted into an artificial bladder; either a loop of ileum used as a conduit with one end opening on the abdominal surface and draining into an ileostomy bag; or implanted into the isolated rectum which then acts as a bladder, and a faecal colostomy is made at the same time.

As primary treatment, these methods have obvious objections, and the treatment of choice should now be regarded as *radical radiation*. This may be either (a) interstitial or (b) external (preferably).
Stage 3. All these are subjects for *external radiation,* the only difficulty at times being the choice between radical and palliative. Radical treatment should be considered if:
1. Growth is still mobile, as assessed on bimanual examination.
2. General condition is good.
3. Age is below 70.
4. Renal function (I.V.P., blood urea) is satisfactory.
If these conditions are not satisfied, radiation should be on a palliative basis.
Stage 4. *Palliative radiation* is the only possibility here. For some advanced cases, particularly in the elderly, the best treatment is no active treatment – beyond sedatives and nursing care.

*Radiation techniques*
1. Interstitial methods include:
    1. Gold grains.
    2. Radium (or cobalt or caesium) needles.
    3. Iridium wire.
These require suprapubic cystotomy.

*Gold grains* are inserted submucosally in one or more rings round and in the tumour (Fig. 9.3). A gold grain magazine-loaded 'gun' is used (Fig. 11.4). These sources have to be specially ordered in advance. The requisite number and strength are worked out after preliminary cystoscopy at which the size of the lesion(s) is estimated. These implants are *permanent,* and remain as foreign bodies in the bladder wall, but very rarely give rise to any complications whatever. They give an effective dose of about 7000 rads.

A radium *needle implant* is possible, but this needs a second operation after a week or so for its removal; this method is therefore hardly ever used now.

An alternative is radioactive *iridium wire* (p. 204) made up into 'hairpin' loops and implanted by a special introducer. The loops are tied by silk threads to an indwelling catheter and withdrawn via the urethra at the end of a week.

Interstitial methods are now giving way to external radiation.
2. External radiation should now always be by megavoltage or cobalt beam. The first step must be the decision between palliative and radical treatment, taking into account the factors listed above under Stage 3, as well as the size and extent of the growth.

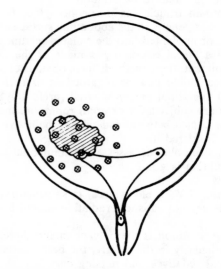

Fig. 9.3 A gold grain implant in the bladder. (*Paterson, Treatment of Malignant Disease by Radiotherapy 2nd edition, Arnold*)

*Radical external radiation* is always a strenuous and trying ordeal for any patient, and is not to be embarked on without full prior assessment and consideration of all the pros and cons.

A typical course takes between three and five weeks, and delivers a tumour dose of 5500-6500 rads. The patient should be in hospital. Careful preliminary radiographic localisation, and full-scale drawing-board planning is carried out (see p. 77). Nurses should attend in the X-ray and physics department to see the detailed preparations for a case. A common technique is a three-field plan similar to Fig. 5.3, p. 77, with one anterior and two postero-lateral oblique fields. Alternatively a rotation technique is good, giving a dosage distribution as in Fig. 9.4.

*Palliative radiation* is very valuable for control of haematuria and pain. Simple technique is indicated, e.g. a parallel pair of anterior and posterior fields giving 3500 rads in 10 sessions, or a rotation method. In practice, about half of all treated bladder cancers are suitable for palliation only.

*Intracavitary* methods have been tried – fluid radioactive isotopes (gold, yttrium) and cytotoxic drugs – but generally given up.

*Nursing and medical care.* Preliminary correction of anaemia and infection is important. The urine is sent for culture and organism sensitivity tests, and the appropriate urinary antiseptic or antibiotic used. The urine should be made sterile if possible before treatment starts, but with an ulcerated mass this may not be possible.

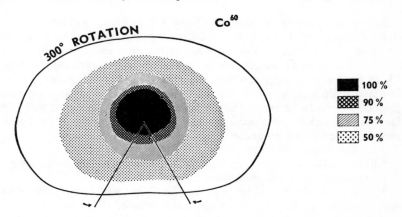

Fig. 9.4 Dose distribution for treatment of bladder by cobalt beam – rotation therapy. Note that the full circle is not used here; 60° at the back are omitted, to decrease dosage to the rectum. (*Paterson, Treatment of Malignant Disease, 2nd edition, Arnold*)

Dysuria and frequency from radiation cystitis during and after the course of radiation are common, but not usually serious unless infection is gross. Painful spasm and strangury may require antispasmodic drugs such as propantheline (Probanthine). Fluid intake must be encouraged, and the effects of radiation cystitis may be reduced by keeping the urine alkaline with oral citrate. Reactions and symptoms may take many weeks to subside. The patient should be warned that he may pass fragments in the urine (blood clot and tumour) and a little blood.

*Late radiation effects.* Late contracture of the bladder and severe telangiectasia with uncontrollable haemorrhage are rare late possibilities. Cystectomy may be indicated.

*Results of radical radiation.* For early cases (Stage 1) the five-year survival is about 75 per cent; for Stage 2 cases 50 per cent; for Stage 3, 20 per cent; and for Stage 4, 10 per cent. The overall figure is about 35 per cent.

*Treatment of recurrences.* After radical radiation, further radiation should never be given – the result would only be a painful necrosis. If total cystectomy is practicable, it should be done. A second palliative course of external radiation may be possible for recurrent symptoms.

*Summary conclusion.* For all except Stage 1 lesions, radiation is now the method of choice, and the results are superior to those of surgery. Interstitial techniques – gold grains, iridium wire – are possible but obsolescent, and the best results come from external megavoltage radiation. Good results are obtained in carefully selected cases, and useful palliation, especially for haematuria, in advanced cases.

## Cancer of the skin

Skin cancers are fairly common (Table 1.2, p. 8) and will form a substantial fraction of the work of a radiotherapy department. Nearly all are treatable as out-patients and the ward nurse may see very few.

Causative factors (sunlight, tar, X-rays, etc.) have been discussed on p. 13. In backward countries, where educational standards are low, extensive and infiltrating growths are seen. Where higher standards prevail, diagnosis tends to be early. Their ready accessibility, combined with the fact that metastasis – if it occurs at all – is generally late, gives most skin cancers an excellent prognosis.

*Types.* The commonest are:

1. Basal cell carcinoma.   2. Squamous carcinoma.   3. Melanoma.

Some rarer types are mentioned below.

1. *Basal cell carcinoma* (or 'Rodent Ulcer') includes 80 per cent of all skin malignancy. It arises from the basal cells of the epidermis. It is probably often caused by strong sunlight, and is particularly common in Australia. Most occur on the face, especially the upper part and around the eyes. There are several clinical types – a raised nodule, a scaly patch, a depressed cicatrising lesion etc. Ulceration is absent at first, but if neglected the lesion will burrow deeply and even erode bone – hence the descriptive term 'rodent'. Exceptionally, e.g. in mental defiiciency, advice is not sought until it has done extensive damage perhaps destroying an eye and eroding the orbit deeply.

Growth is slow, and they may exist for years with only very gradual increase in size, but superficial ulceration, scabbing and bleeding are usually early. A history of a year or two is common. They do not metastasise, but at a late stage they can turn into squamous epithelioma and then give rise to secondaries.

*Treatment.* Small lesions are easily excised and this is satisfactory treatment. But recurrence is common, as surgeons tend to be conservative in facial lesions. On the eyelids and nose, excision may involve difficult plastic repair – which is rarely justified, as radiation generally gives good results. Cure should be achieved in 95 per cent of cases.

If bone is involved, radiation may be used first, followed by complete excision and repair, since radiation is unlikely to deal satisfactorily with invaded bone. If cartilage is invaded – pinna or ala nasi – surgery is again preferable, as the avascularity of cartilage makes for poor healing or necrosis.

2. *Squamous carcinoma* (epithelioma) is the next commonest. The history is shorter – weeks or months. It can occur anywhere on the body surface, but the face is the commonest site.

*Treatment.* Surgery is again satisfactory, especially for small lesions. Healing after simple excision will take a shorter time than a full-scale radiation reaction, and may be preferable for this reason, especially on parts of the body other than the face. Impaired blood supply is another reason for preferring surgery – e.g. in presence of varicose ulceration or chronic radio-dermatitis. Many cases – and in many centres, most cases – are treated by radiation, and the end results for early cases are nearly as good as for basal cell lesions.

Lymph-node metastasis is infrequent, but must be looked for, and suspicious nodes should be treated surgically if possible.

3. *Melanoma.* This is a very common and usually innocent tumour, associated with the pigment melanin. The name means 'black' or 'dark' (Greek) and is given to the pigmented flat spots or raised moles which most people have, usually as birthmarks, of light to dark brown colour.

The name 'naevus' (Latin for 'mole') is also used, but this is unfortunate, as the same word is also applied to the angioma (a tumour of blood vessels). Since melanomas are associated developmentally with nervous tissue, the terms 'neuro-naevus' and 'angio-naevus' are preferable.

Malignant change is uncommon, but should be suspected if a melanoma increases in size, darkens in colour, ulcerates or bleeds. Malignant melanoma can also arise from pigment cells (melanoblasts) in previously normal skin. It is also called 'melano-carcinoma'.

They are the most treacherous and dangerous of all skin cancers. Spread is by lymphatics at first to regional nodes and often to adjacent skin areas, later via the bloodstream to lungs, liver etc.

*Treatment* should always be by wide surgical excision if possible, since their radiosensitivity is usually low. On the limbs, perfusion with a cytotoxic drug may be valuable (see pp. 228-9).

*Radiation techniques.* Several methods are available, all giving good results, including:

1. Radium (or one of its substitutes, e.g. cobalt) – surface mould or implant.

2. Gold grains – surface mould or implant.

3. X-rays – usually at low voltage, as great penetration is not required; in fact it would be a positive disadvantage. Voltages in the region of 50-100 kV are most commonly used (Fig. 4.14, p. 57).

*Radium mould.* Surface radium is popular at some centres, while in others it has been given up. Figure 9.5 illustrates the general principle. The radioactive sources are mounted on the surface of the mould, usually some plastic material carefully shaped on a plaster-cast model of the part. The patient must, of course, be in hospital during treatment, which takes about a week. The mould is carefully fitted and strapped on to the part, and is worn for periods of 8-12 hr per day. It is taken off at night and kept in the radium safe.

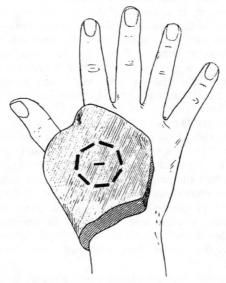

Fig. 9.5 Diagram of radium (or cobalt etc.) sources, mounted on a surface mould, for treating an epithelioma on the back of the hand. (*Paterson, Treatment of Malignant Disease, 2nd edition, Arnold*)

Radium moulds involve highly skilled preparation, occupation of a hospital bed, and increased radiation background in the ward – all of which are reasons for their obsolescence, since X-rays almost always give equally good results.

*Gold grain mould.* This does not involve hospital admission and is particularly useful for an aged patient at home. Figure 9.6 illustrates the method. Adhesive elastoplast felt is used, and the sources arranged to be at about 0.5 cm from the skin surface. After the treatment time – about one week – the patient is instructed to remove the mould and either burn it or return it to hospital for recovery of the gold or other precious metal. Even if the mould is lost, the rapid decay of radioactivity will forestall any radiation hazard.

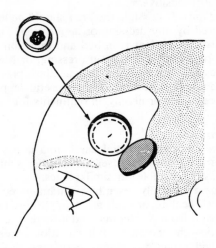

Fig. 9.6 Mould applied to a skin cancer. A ring of felt 0.5 in thick surrounds the projecting tumour. A circle of zinc oxide dressing carrying the sources is mounted on the ring, and covered by another layer of dressing. *(Paterson, Treatment of Malignant Disease, 2nd edition, Arnold)*

*Superficial X-rays* are by far the most popular and important technique. In a typical case, this means out-patient attendance at 8-10 sessions, either daily or on alternate days. Five-hundred rads are given each time, to a total of 4000-5000 rads. This is followed by erythema and dry or moist peeling as described on p. 58. Treatment of the reaction is on the lines laid down on pp. 90-92.

Fractionation of dosage is desirable, but for small lesions – up to about 2 cm – a single shot of about 2000 rads may be given. This is useful, e.g. for elderly patients or those with long distances to travel, but the cosmetic results are less good and the risk of late necrosis is increased.

Late skin changes (atrophy, pigmentation etc.) may appear and are unpredictable, though not usually serious. But if appearances are important – especially in younger women – operation by a plastic surgeon may be preferable for cosmetic reasons.

Lesions on the eyelids are fairly common – especially basal cell lesions at the medial ends near the bridge of the nose (inner canthus). When X-ray treatment is given, it is important to protect the cornea and lens. A small eye-shield, incorporating about 1 mm thickness of lead, is inserted beneath the eyelid(s) like a contact lens, after anaesthetising the conjunctival surface. After treatment sterile liquid paraffin may be instilled and the eye covered with a pad. The patient is instructed to retain this for a few hours, in case particles of grit etc. enter the eye and damage the cornea while it is still insensitive.

*Treatment of reactions.* If possible the area should be left alone and undisturbed, uncovered by any dressing or application. This is practicable for small areas or if the patient is in bed and infection can be avoided. Otherwise simple tulle gras with a plain dressing, or Melolin, is enough. Greasy substances like vaseline are bad as they prevent natural discharges and encourage infection. Other useful applications are — calamine cream; cetrimide or neomycin ointments for infection (see also p. 91-92).

## Other skin tumours

*Bowen's disease* or intra-epithelial carcinoma is a superficial lesion, often multiple, on the trunk and elsewhere, rather similar to basal cell carcinoma and easily treatable on similar lines.

*Kerato-acanthoma* clinically resembles squamous epithelioma, but is benign and often self-healing, or heals after simple curettage. Even biopsy may not distinguish it from carcinoma, and if there is doubt, it should be treated as squamous carcinoma by full radiation or excision.

Sweat glands and sebaceous glands may give rise to *adenoma* or *adenocarcinoma*, and these are best excised.

*Secondary carcinoma* often appears as nodules just beneath the epidermis, especially from a lung primary, or in the skin flaps after mastectomy. Local X-ray treatment is useful for temporary control and to prevent fungation.

*Reticulosis.* Skin lesions may be an early manifestation of lympho-reticular disease. The most serious is mycosis fungoides (see p. 181).

*Summary conclusion.* For the commonest skin cancers — basal cell and squamous epitheliomas — radiation is generally a very good alternative to surgery and is widely used as the first line of treatment. Surgery is available if radiation fails.

For malignant melanoma, surgery is always preferable, if practicable.

## Some special sites

*Lip.* Excellent results are usually achieved by radation, which is the method of choice in most cases. X-rays are satisfactory, but some prefer a 'sandwich mould' of radium as in Fig. 9.7. The functional results are better than those of surgery, which can be reserved for radiation failures or recurrences.

*Penis.* Cancer never occurs in males circumcised in infancy. Hygienic factors are therefore important. (See also p. 31 for relevance in cancer of cervix.)

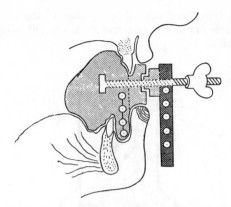

Fig. 9.7 A double lip mould. Must be made individually to fit the patient. The tongue is pushed as far as possible away from the radium sources. (*Paterson, 'Treatment of Malignant Disease', 2nd edition, Arnold*)

Many cases occur in the elderly. Where expectation of life is anyhow not long, and especially if the growth is infiltrating the glans or shaft deeply, surgery is shorter and safer. For younger men with localised growths, X-ray therapy is preferable for psychological reasons and can be curative. Later surgery can be used in cases of failure. Circumcision should be carried out first, followed by a 4-5 week course of radiotherapy – kilovoltage and megavoltage are equally satisfactory. Secondary inguinal nodes should be treated surgically if possible.

*Vulva.* Epithelioma is best treated by excision, since this region is intolerant of high radiation dosage. If surgery is ruled out for any reason, a radium needle implant is a possible alternative and can be successful in growths of limited extent.

## Cancer of the testis

This is another field where radiation has an important, even decisive, part to play, in combination with surgery.

The commonest cancers are:

(a) seminoma;    (b) teratoma.

Much rarer is choriocarcinoma in some ways analogous to the choriocarcinoma of the placenta (p. 232).

Primary treatment is by *orchidectomy* and the exact histology is determined by microscopy.

As always, it is important to secure all possible information about the extent of spread. Figure 9.8 shows the routes of lymphatic extension. The most important area of lymph-node metastasis is the central retro-peritoneal abdominal strip – the *paraortic nodes*. Pelvic nodes may also be involved. At the time of orchidectomy, careful examination of the abdomen under general anaesthesia should be made to detect secondary masses. Further lymphatic spread is upward to the mediastinum, and even to supraclavicular nodes (especially on the left side) which should always be palpated.

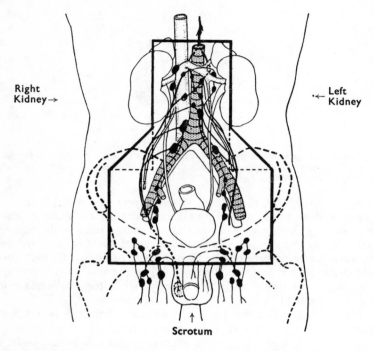

Right Kidney→

←Left Kidney

↑
Scrotum

Fig. 9.8 Lymphatic drainage of testis and outline of polygonal megavoltage field to include nodes of groins, pelvis and paraortic area. Scrotum and other testis not included in the field. (*Raven, Cancer, Vol. 5, Butterworths*)

Routinely a chest film is taken for possible mediastinal and pulmonary secondaries, and intravenous pyelography done, both to outline the position of the kidneys (see below) and to detect any deviation of the ureters by secondary masses.

Lymphangiography should also be carried out if possible (see p.176).

1. *Seminoma.* Following orchidectomy, it is essential to irradiate the retro-peritoneal lymphatic regions whether there is evidence of spread or not, since microscopic secondary deposits, which cannot be demonstrated clinically or radiologically, are common.

The area is extensive, and if the growth were squamous carcinoma, it would be impossible to give an adequate cancericidal dose − over 5000 rads − to such a large volume, because of the inevitable damage to bowel. However, seminoma happens to be the *most radiosensitive of all epithelial cancers,* and a dose of about 3000 rads is usually curative. It is quite practicable to give this relatively moderate dose to the large abdominal volume, and the results are usually good. Figure 9.8 shows the simple radiation technique – two large specially shaped fields at megavoltage, anterior and posterior, to include the pelvis and most of the abdomen. The exact size and shape of the fields will be determined by the findings – e.g. if there are palpable or demonstrable masses in the kidney region, they will have to be covered. It is very important, however, to ensure that the kidneys (or at least one kidney) do not receive more than 2000 rads, otherwise fatal radiation nephritis is a likely consequence (see p. 96). The dose is given by daily fractionation over 4-5 weeks and the general upset is rarely severe.

Some workers routinely include the other testis in the radiation field, to be on the safe side. The consequences – i.e. permanent sterility, but not impotence – must be explained to the patient in advance. Even if the testis is not inside the field, it will receive about 200 rads from scattered megavoltage radiation. This will not sterilise, but could cause gene mutations. If the patient already has a family, it is a good alternative to sterilise him by vasectomy, to exclude any genetic complications. If he is young and wishes to retain the possibility of a family, the radiation should be at 250 kV and the testicle enclosed during treatment in a lead chamber one cm thick. This will prevent the testis receiving more than 10 rads, an acceptable dose.

This combined scheme of treatment – primary surgery plus radiation to lymph-nodes – gives very good results. If disease is clinically limited to the testis, the *five-year survival is nearly 90 per cent,* and even in the presence of demonstrable abdominal secondaries it is over 60 per cent. This compares with 25 per cent for early cases in the days before radiotherapy.

Even mediastinal and pulmonary involvement is not hopeless, and treatment to the chest is usually practicable and can be curative.

*Cytotoxic* therapy is also now being used for disseminated seminoma, e.g. melphalan. It is also used prophylactically after radiation, to deal with possible micro-metastases.

2. *Teratoma.* Here the situation is unfortunately different, since radiosensitivity, though variable, is usually low. If radiation to the lymphatic areas is attempted at all, the dose has to be as high as possible, at least 4500 rads, and this is verging on the danger line. Some therapists therefore prefer to rely on *cytotoxic drug therapy,* using combination of vinblastine, actinomycin-D and adriamycin.

For the earliest stage of teratoma, i.e. all investigations for spread negative, it is reasonable to withhold further therapy and leave on observation only, since 75 per cent of these will never need further treatment.

*Summary conclusion.* For most testicular cancer, especially seminoma, the treatment of choice is surgery for the primary (orchidectomy) and radiation for secondary nodes. The results for seminoma are outstandingly good.

## Cancer of the prostate

Cancer of the prostate gland, situated just below the base of the bladder, is a common disease of elderly men. After lung and bowel it is the next most frequent fatal cancer, and accounts for 7 per cent of all male cancer deaths.

*Pathology.* Almost all are adenocarcinoma. Direct spread is to the bladder and rectum, then to other pelvic tissues. Lymph spread is to pelvic and paraortic nodes, and sometimes to the inguinal group in the groin. It readily invades pelvic veins and thence to pelvic bones and vertebrae. Bone secondaries are often of sclerotic type, showing an increased density in the radiograph instead of the usual bone erosion.

The prostate has analogies with the breast and is under hormonal control. Removal of male hormone by orchidectomy, or administration of female hormones (oestrogens), causes shrinkage of the normal gland, and often of cancerous prostatic growth also.

The gland secretes an enzyme – acid phosphatase – which can be estimated in the blood. Abnormally large amounts may be found in many cases of prostatic cancer, especially if there are widespread metastases. This is useful in diagnosis.

Early cancer is not uncommonly found unexpectedly on histological examination of prostates removed for benign enlargement.

*Treatment.* Radical prostatectomy is ideal but only a very small fraction are suitable. Most patients are unfit for major surgery, and early diagnosis before dissemination in anyhow rare. Such patients are best managed by hormonal methods. Most tumours regress on administration of oestrogens (e.g. Stilboestrol). Side effects may follow oestrogen therapy – nausea, enlargement of breasts, atrophy of testes, pigmentation of nipples.

(It is of historical interest that this was the first clinical application of hormonal cancer control – by Huggins of Chicago in 1941. He was later awarded a Nobel prize.)

The beneficial effects on primary and secondaries may be prolonged, even several years, but the growth eventually escapes from control. When this occurs, or if oestrogens fail, improvement may be obtainable by removing the source of male hormones, by operative removal of the testes (bilateral orchidectomy). Further details on hormones are in Ch. 12.

If urinary obstruction persists, TUR, (trans-urethral resection), to remove the offending part of the prostate, is indicated. In this operation the instruments are passed by the surgeon along the urethra, and portions of the prostate are scoooped out with a cutting edge.

Painful bone secondaries may be irradiated, e.g. to 3000 rads in two weeks, but results are less reliable than in breast cancer. For widespread bone deposits, pain may be relieved for many months by intravenous injection of radioactive phosphorus (P-32). The tumour tissue causes a regenerative reaction in adjacent bone, with increased metabolic turnover – hence the increased selective uptake of phosphorus – (the mechanism is the basis of isotope bone scans).

*Radiation* to the prostate itself gave such poor results in previous years (orthovoltage, radium needles, infiltration with radio-gold, etc.) that it was largely abandoned, and prostatic cancer was considered insufficiently response to be worth attempts at radical radiotherapy.

Megavoltage is still not widely used with radical intent, but has proved capable of achieving local control in a proportion of inoperable cases, so that it is now coming into use and giving useful results with improved technique. Technique and dosage may be similar to that for bladder cancer (see above). Localisation is assisted by contrast medium in both bladder and rectum. The best results come from small – volume technique, with fields about 7 × 7 cm, delivering about 7500 rads in about $7\frac{1}{2}$ weeks. Since the rectum is immediately adjacent, it must share in the high dosage. Rectal reactions will inevitably occur, and the risk of occasional serious damage has to be accepted.

*Prognosis.* The natural history of prostatic cancer tends to be long. The average five-year survival is about 40 per cent. If there are no distant metastases, hormonal management alone is capable of achieving this. The rare eases of operability do better, but if there are secondaries at the time of diagnosis, survival is only about 20 per cent.

### Tumours of bone

Primary malignant growths of bone are:

*Osteosarcoma* (osteogenic sarcoma). *Chondrosarcoma.*

*Fibrosarcoma.*                       *Chordoma.*

*Osteoclastoma* (giant-cell tumour) is in a class apart – usually benign, occasionally malignant.

The following occur in bone, but arise in bone marrow and/or reticular tissue:

*Myeloma* – see p. 186-7.

*Ewing's tumour.* – see p. 187-8.

*Reticulum cell sarcoma* and other reticuloses.

*Malignant granuloma.*

These are often listed under Bone tumours for convenience.

*Secondary growths* in bone. These are the commonest of all malignant lesions involving bone.

### Osteosarcoma

This is the most common and most malignant primary bone cancer. Most occur in young people, in the second decade, and involve mainly the femur, tibia or humerus.

Osteosarcoma is radio-resistant, and the obvious and logical treatment is immediate primary amputation. However, the results are so poor, only about 10 per cent surviving five years becuase of the very high incidence of lung secondaries, that many orthopaedic surgeons have abandoned this form of treatment as it tends to give the patient the worst of both worlds, i.e. loss of a limb without saving of life.

A useful compromise is to radiate the tumour first to hold it in check, while the patient is observed and serial chest films taken. Most of the cases that are doomed to develop lung secondaries will have shown up within seven months or so. For those who survive longer with no signs of metastasis, amputation of the primary can then be undertaken, with greatly improved chances of success.

Since the tumour is radio-resistant, high dosage is needed. High energy radiation is used, giving 1000 rads per week to a total of about 7000 rads or even higher. Even with this regime, the five-year survival is not much above 20 per cent, but it can spare many patients the misery of superfluous amputation. Total destruction of the local tumour can be achieved in about a third of treated cases, and there is a strong temptation to postpone amputation as long as the lesion is quiescent. This is not in the patient's best interest, especially in the lower limb, where a good prosthesis is practicable, but has more justification in the upper limb, where amputation is particularly hard to advise.

If the growth is in an inoperable situation, e.g. spine, we have to depend on radiation, for growth restraint at least, and a faint hope of permanent control.

If pain is severe, or fungation occurs, amputation may be necessary as a palliative measure, even in the presence of known secondaries.

*Chemotherapy* is now on trial as a supplement to surgery. In the last few years, combination chemotherapy with vincristine and cyclophosphamide has produced temporary responses visible in the chest film. More aggressive chemotherapy is by high-dose methotrexate with folinic acid rescue to prevent severe toxic side-effects (see p. 225). Other drugs in use are: adriamycin and melphalan. This therapy aims at destroying metastatic cells at the microscopic stage, and is started soon after amputation. The early results are encouraging, but insufficient time has elapsed for proper assessment.

*Osteosarcoma on Paget's disease of bone.* There is a second peak of incidence in the elderly, where bone sarcoma may develop on a basis of Paget's disease. The prognosis is virtually hopeless with any form of treatment, but radiation may relieve symptoms.

*Chondrosarcoma and fibrosarcoma.* Primary surgery is always the treatment of choice if possible. If not, radiation may provide a measure of temporary growth restraint and relief of symptoms.

*Chordoma.* This is a rare tumour, arising from remnants of the embryonic notochord (Greek 'noton' = back), a cartilaginous band forming the basis of the spinal column. The commonest sites are the ends, i.e. base of skull and sacro-coccygeal region. Complete surgical removal is rarely possible. Radical radiation to tolerance dosage may hold it in check for prolonged periods.

*Osteoclastoma* (giant cell tumour of bone). This is an uncommon and peculiar tumour, mostly in young adults. Most are benign, but some are sarcomatous, either from the start or in the course of years. Radiation can give excellent results, but because of their liability to treacherous behaviour, surgery is safer unless the site is inoperable.

*Reticulo-sarcoma.* This may be solitary or part of a generalised reticulosis. They are locally curable with moderate doses.

*Granuloma.* There is a rather obscure group of lesions, sometimes labelled Histiocytosis-X, of doubtful pathology, possibly metabolic disorders, and usually occurring in the younger age group. The one most likely to be seen in a radiotherapy department is the *eosinophil granuloma* which presents as a tumour in bone, often solitary but sometimes multiple. It tends to recur after curettage, but responds well to low doses of radiation, about 1000-1500 rads.

## Bone secondaries

A radiotherapy ward is never long without one or more of these, the commonest bone tumour of all. The most frequent primary sites are – breast, lung, prostate, kidney and thyroid – i.e. mostly adenocarcinomas. The metastatic deposits come via the bloodstream, and this means that the growth is already disseminated, often widely, and the ultimate prognosis almost always very poor, though great relief is possible for months and even years.

The usual *clinical presentation* is pain, caused by tension of the periosteum or pressure on nerve roots as they emerge from the spinal canals (Fig. 9.9). *Early diagnosis* is important, before bone destruction has advanced far enough to cause pathological fracture or compression paraplegia. X-ray films may show the deposits, usually as osteolytic (i.e. bone-destroying) rarefactions, but sometimes as patches of increased density or sclerosis (especially in prostatic cancer, also in breast cancer at times).

But a secondary deposit, e.g. in a vertebral body must be of some size – about 2 cm – before it will show up in a film. If we have a patient with a known primary liable to bony secondaries, such as breast cancer clinical suspicion alone will usually justify local X-ray therapy on the reasonable assumption that secondaries are responsible.

In the *routine investigation* of many types of cancer, skeletal X-ray surveys may be made – either complete, or of spine, ribs and pelvis – but unsuspected findings of silent secondaries are very uncommon. A more searching method is now available in the *radioactive bone scan* (see p. 52) which can show up secondaries many months before the stage of possible radiological diagnosis. These scans are now being undertaken in some centres as the (expensive) equipment becomes more widely available. The finding of latent secondaries will obviously affect the whole treatment plan and prognosis.

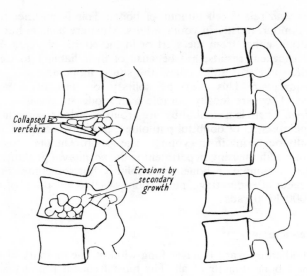

Fig. 9.9 Diagrammatic radiological appearances of normal spinal column and secondary deposits from cancer (e.g. breast).

*Treatment* of diagnosed deposits will depend on the total situation:

a. What is the local condition of the bone? – is it considerably eroded? – is there a pathological fracture present or impending?

b. Is it a solitary secondary (as far as can be determined) or are there widespread deposits, bony and/or visceral?

c. What is the patient's age, general condition, and reasonable expectation of remaining life?

d. Is the growth hormone dependent, and if so, what part can hormone therapy play?

As a rule, the urgent primary objective is *relief of pain,* and for this radiation is usually the method of choice. In most cases the symptomatic results are most gratifying. This palliative role of radiotherapy is one of its great historic triump h and would alone justify the installation of an expensive unit. For a case like that of Fig. 9.10, a single field, either deep therapy or high energy, suffices, giving about 2000 rads in 4-5 days (Fig. 8.6, p. 122). For a limb a simple parallel pair of fields is used.

If *pathological fracture* of a long bone has occurred – e.g. femur or humerus – operative internal fixation of the fragments by an intra-medullary metal pin will give immediate relief and allow early mobilisation. The deposit can then be irradiated to destroy the growth locally.

For an elderly patient with widespread involvement from e.g. lung cancer, simple pain relief and general nursing care will contribute to a peaceful passage. But for a middle-aged woman with bone secondaries from breast cancer, even if multiple, good management, using a combination of local X-rays and general hormone therapy, may often keep her alive and fit for many years, e.g. oophorectomy, adrenalectomy etc. (see pp. 207-13). Similar management for prostatic cancer with oestrogens, orchidectomy and local X-ray therapy also gives good results.

If it involves a weight-bearing bone such as the femur, a longer course – e.g. 3500 rads in two weeks – may lead to good re-calcification and allow weight-bearing again in 2-3 months. But if bone deposits are widespread and hormonal improvement is not applicable, treatment should be confined to the painful areas only, because attempts to irradiate many bones will exhaust the limited marrow tolerance still left. For such cases *single shot therapy*, giving 1000-1500 rads in one session, is simple and easy for the patient, and can give good relief.

*The nursing care* of these patients is important and can be difficult. The risk of pathological fracture must always be kept in mind and forestalled – or dealt with if it has occurred – by use of plaster shells, fracture boards, arm slings and pillows, plastic neck collars etc. If plaster slabs or shells are used, it may be advisable to cut large holes in them for the X-ray treatment fields. If the ends of the fragments after pathological fracture override, orthopaedic traction with a Thomas's splint and Balkan frame may be needed. The splint may have to be removed at each treatment session, though it may be possible to wheel the whole bed to the X-ray treatment room without disturbing the patient.

Lesions of the spine, especially with paraplegia, are particularly difficult, and nursing skills will be fully taxed. Attention to skin and pressure points is important, especially if they have to be irradiated, and baby powder or silicone cream should be used instead of ordinary talcum (see p. 91). Ripple beds are valuable, as are non-adhesive dressings (e.g. Melolin) for ulcerated areas. When orthopaedic and radiation treatments are over, physiotherapy and rehabilitation, aided by spinal corsets, walking calipers etc., are begun.

## Cancers of connective tissues

These include various sarcomas:

*Fibrosarcoma* (fibrous tissue). *Myosarcoma* (muscle – including leiomyosarcoma and rhabdomyosarcoma, of smooth and striped muscle respectively). *Liposarcoma* (fat). *Synovial sarcoma* (synovial membrane lining joints, tendon sheaths etc.).

They are all *resistant to radiation,* and should always be treated surgically if possible, though they tend to recur locally. If unsuitable for surgery, there may be a useful palliative response with growth restraint from radiation.

*Malignant synovioma* (synovial sarcoma) is a possible exception, since it may respond to high dosage, like some cases of osteosarcoma.

## Cancer of the ovary

Ovarian cancer accounts for about 5 per cent of cancer in women. Most ovarian tumours are benign, but one in five are malignant – especially after the menopause, when the proportion rises to a half. There is a bewildering variety of histological types, but the great majority are adenocarcinoma and cystic – i.e. *cystadenocarcinoma* (subdivided into serous and mucinous types).

Growth is unfortunately insidious and clinically silent for a long time, until pressure symptoms occur – abdominal swelling, pain, dysuria.

*Treatment* is always primarily *surgical* if possible, and it is only at laparotomy that the full extent of spread can be assessed. It may involve one ovary or both; tubes and uterus may be invaded, and there may be spread to other pelvic organs directly or via lymphatics to paraortic lymph-nodes (as in seminoma testis – Fig. 9.8, p. 164). Multiple peritoneal and omental nodules may be found, and more or less fluid exudate, often blood-stained.

*Radical surgery,* with removal of ovaries and uterus, is actually feasible only in about 30 per cent. If growth appears localised and surgical removal seems complete, no further treatment is indicated, and the prognosis in well-differentiated histological types is fairly good.

If the growth is anaplastic, *post-operative radiation* may be considered. If the surgeon is doubtful about the completeness of his operation – e.g. if there has been rupture of a malignant cyst with spill into the peritoneal cavity, or if there is undoubted growth that had to be left behind – the case is commonly referred for radiotherapy.

Even if complete removal is clearly impossible, as much as possible of the growth should still be removed surgically, to leave a smaller residue for post-operative therapy, which can give prolonged palliation.

If the residue appears limited to the pelvis, external megavoltage radiation may be given, up to 5000 rads in four weeks. The highest tolerable dose is needed, since the radiosensitivity of most growths is not high. High doses carry some definite risk of morbidity and late complications (see p. 92), especially as there is very likely to be some bowel adherent in the operation field, but this risk must be accepted if there seems to be no chance of success without further treatment.

Lymph-node metastases are common, and some therapists therefore enlarge the fields upwards to include the paraortic region (as in Fig. 9.8). This increase in volume involves a lowering of the tolerable radiation dosage, and an increased liability to radiation reactions. Diarrhoea, sickness etc. may occur – these effects and their treatment are described on pp. 92-93.

If there are widespread abdominal deposits, external radiation is probably useless. If the general condition is poor, it is better to withold radiation entirely.

If there has been spill of potential seedlings in the peritoneal cavity at operation, some workers advise instillation of a radioactive isotope or *cytotoxic drug* intraperitoneally, to destroy microscopic deposits before they can take root (see pp. 201-2, 227-8).

*Value of post-operative radiation.* This is difficult to assess. Whether it lengthens life is doubtful, and inoperable growths are probably really incurable. But it can certainly improve the quality of life by controlling symptoms.

*Cytotoxic drugs.* For advanced cases, there is now a tendency to replace – or supplement – radiation by a cytotoxic drug. The most favoured are chlorambucil, thiotepa and cyclophosphamide, and good palliative results can undoubtedly be achieved in many cases (see Ch. 13).

*Ascites.* Malignant peritoneal effusions are common and distressing. Repeated tappings are exhausting for the patient, and the loss of protein debilitating. External radiation is of no value, but useful results can be obtained in 50 per cent of cases by instillation into the peritoneal cavity of either a cytotoxic drug or a radioactive isotope.

Some special varieties of ovarian growths are worth mentioning:

1. *Pseudomucinous cystadenoma* – usually technically benign, though a few are adenocarcinomatous. The peculiar jelly-like material in the cysts can be most troublesome if the cyst ruptures and deposits seedlings on the peritoneal surfaces. Intra-peritoneal infusion of radio-gold or yttrium may kill these off, but if recurrence occurs, no treatment seems to be of value short of laparotomy and manual removal of the material.

2. *Dysgerminoma.* This is a rare tumour, often in young women or children, but of interest to the radiotherapist, as it is analogous to seminoma testis in the male. It is therefore very radiosensitive and can be successfully treated by similar large fields to include lymph-nodes (Fig. 9.8).

3. *Granulosa cell tumour.* These secrete ovarian hormone, causing uterine hyperplasia and bleeding. They are of variable malignancy, from benign to aggressive. Late recurrence can occur after many years. Radiation may be valuable post-operatively.

# 10. Lympho-reticular Disorders

*Any man's death diminishes me
because I am involved in mankind.
And therefore never send to know
for whom the bell tolls;
It tolls for thee.*

John Donne

This is a diverse group, to which the name 'Reticulosis' is also applied.

## Malignant lymphomas

The term lymphoma is now used to include all the primary malignancies of lymph nodes. A simple classification, and in order of frequency, is as follows:

1. *Hodgkin's disease*
2. *Lymphosarcoma*

This includes a wide spectrum of malignancy ranging from well differentiated *lymphocytic lymphoma* to undifferentiated (or lymphoblastic) lymphoma.

3. *Reticulum cell sarcoma*

The modern name for reticulum cell is 'histiocyte', hence the alternative name – *histiocytic lymphoma*.

4. *Follicular lymphoma*

This used to be (and still may be) called *giant follicular lymphoma*.

Modern pathologists classify lymphomas not only according to the cell type but also by the tissue pattern. The cells may either form a diffuse sheet or be arranged in nodules which resemble normal lymphoid follicles. Most of the above types can therefore be subdivided into *diffuse* or *nodular* types. The diffuse is more anaplastic and of worse prognosis than the nodular.

The various types show clinical as well as histological differences, especially in regard to prognosis and survival. But they also have many similarities, so that some general statements can be made covering all or most of them:

a. A common presentation is node enlargement in a single focus, especially in the neck, and other groups appear to follow by spread from the first. Other cases seem to be of multifocal origin, i.e. to arise at several sites simultaneously.

b. These foci almost always respond well to treatment at first, but a time may come (if primary treatment fails) when widespread deposits are present, including bone marrow. Lesions may eventually become refractory to treatment and the patient succumbs to exhaustion and infection.

c. Progress of disease is often slow, and patients may do well for many years.

d. The role of surgery was, till recently, restricted mainly to node biopsy, but is now assuming greater importance, especially in Hodgkin's disease, for laparotomy, etc.

e. Radiation is a major part of the management of most cases, especially in the earlier stages while disease is still confined to lymphoid tissue.

f. Radiation is usually by large fields, in some form of regional therapy, to include large blocks of lymphatic tissue.

g. Cytotoxic chemotherapy is now of major importance, and often the chief or even the sole weapon in later stages when disease has spread beyond lymphoid tissues.

## Hodgkin's disease

Thomas Hodgkin (1798-1866), a physician at Guy's Hospital, London, was the first to describe it. Alternative names are lymphadenoma or lymphogranuloma.

*Clinical features.* The first symptom is usually painless enlargement of a group of nodes, particularly in the neck, but sometimes in axilla or inguinal region. In some cases mediastinal or abdominal nodes may enlarge first, causing cough, dyspnoea or pain in the chest or abdomen. The spleen may be palpably enlarged. Later spread to extra-lymphatic tissues may involve almost any organ − liver, bone, central nervous system, skin, etc., with a variety of associated symptoms (jaundice, nerve palsies, etc.). General symptoms include − malaise, loss of weight, tiredness, pruritus (itching − often wrongly spelled 'pruritis'), sweats (especially at night). There may be a characteristic type of fever (Pel-Ebstein fever, after the workers who first described it), in waves lasting a week or two, separated by afebrile intervals.

A peculiar symptom, of unknown cause, is severe pain in nodes, etc. after taking even small quantities of alcohol.

*Investigations.* The first step is usually node biopsy, to establish the diagnosis and histological type. To enable vital decisions on treatment to be made, it is essential to obtain as much information as possible on the extent of involvement (Staging). Some or all of the following investigations should be carried out:

Full blood count including E.S.R. (erythrocyte sedimentation rate);
Chest X-ray;
Lymphangiography and I.V.P.;
Bone marrow biopsy;

Isotope scan of liver and spleen;

Laparotomy

*Lymphangiography* (or *lymphography*) came into use in the late 1950s. A blue dye is injected intradermally between the toes on the dorsum of each foot. Movement and massage assist its take-up by lymphatic vessels which are thus made visible. A lymphatic trunk is exposed by dissection (under local anaesthesia) and a radio-opaque contrast medium (similar to that used in pyelography) is injected. It passes along the vessels of the limb, to successive groups of nodes. Enlarged nodes with irregular 'moth-eaten' patches due to malignant deposits can be demonstrated. But if the whole node has been replaced by malignant tissue, the lymphatic entry will be completely blocked and the node will not show up at all.

This technique has opened up the pelvic and paraortic nodes to inspection. Normally any enlargement cannot be detected by palpation till the node mass is huge. Now we can examine the state of the nodes in the early stages, and this information is of immense value in improving our assessment and management. It is unfortunately not possible to visualise mediastinal nodes in the same way. After a lymphogram, the contrast medium remains visible in the nodes for up to 18 months, and follow-up radiographs are valuable in detecting enlargement at an early stage.

I.V.P. should follow lymphography. This will provide evidence of renal function and the position of the ureters will be another indicator. One or both may be displaced and so provide indirect evidence of node masses which have not taken up the radio-opaque lymphographic contrast medium and so cannot be directly visualised.

Isotope scan of liver and spleen will reveal the size of the spleen even if it is not palpable, and may show 'cold' areas in the liver suggestive of malignant deposits.

Surgical *laparotomy* is advisable in many cases, as shown in Table 10.1. This is a drastic step, involving some morbidity and even occasional mortality − a high price to pay. The justification for this lies in the vital importance of finding out the precise state of affairs inside the abdomen, since the optimum line of treatment (radiation or drugs) will depend on this information, and there is no other means of getting it. The surgeon removes the spleen (splenectomy) which is sent to the pathologist for microscopy. He also examines the paraortic and other node areas, and takes one or more nodes for biopsy; the lymphographic picture may help to guide him to suspicious nodes. The liver surface is also inspected and biopsies are taken of liver tissue and any other suspicious masses found. Before laparotomy, a case might appear to be early − Stage I or II (see below) − with nodes above the diaphragm. If abdominal involvement is discovered, the stage is changed to III, or even IV if liver biopsy is positive − and this will change the whole scheme of treatment. It is in any event advantageous to remove the spleen, since clinicial assessment is grossly fallacious. If it is not palpable clinically, many are nevertheless found to be invaded; and surgery is a much more efficient way of dealing with an involved spleen than radiation.

*Histological type.* It is important to determine the histological type, from the node biopsy. Four groups are recognised, and they have great prognostic significance. From most favourable to least favourable they are:

| Lymphocytic predominance | (LP) |
| Nodular sclerosing | (NS) |
| Mixed cellularity | (MC) |
| Lymphocytic depletion | (LD) |

*Staging* is of fundamental importance:

Stage I. Limited to one group of lymph nodes.

Stage II. Two or more groups of nodes, all on the same side of the diaphragm.

Stage III. Disease on both sides of the diaphragm, but not extending beyond the lympho-reticular system.

Stage IV. Disease extending beyond the lymphoreticular system (e.g. liver, bone, skin, etc.)

'Lympho-reticular system' includes lymphnodes, spleen and Waldeyer's ring (i.e. the broken ring of lymphoid tissue at the entrance to the pharynx, comprising the faucial, lingual and pharyngeal tonsils).

All stages are also subclassified into A or B:

A – general symptoms absent.

B – general symptoms present – especially fever and weight loss; pruritus and night sweats are less important and by themselves do not signify a B.

Table 10.1 Management of Hodgkins disease

| Clinical Stage | Histological type | Laparotomy | Treatment |
| --- | --- | --- | --- |
| IA, IIA | Nodular sclerosis<br>Lymphocyte predominance | No | Radiotherapy –<br>Mantle or inverted Y |
| IA, IIA | Mixed cell<br>Lymphocyte depletion | Yes | Radiotherapy –<br>Mantle plus inverted Y<br>(= TNI) |
| IB, IIB, IIIA | All types | Yes | Radiotherapy<br>TNI |
| IIIB, IV | All types | No | Combination<br>chemotherapy |

*Treatment*

Up to the 1960's textbooks of medicine stated that Hodgkin's disease was invariably fatal. *Modern radiotherapy – and now chemotherapy – have revolutionised treatment and prognosis.*

Table 10.1 summarises current methods and indications for the various histological types and clinical stages.

*Radiation technique.* The general rule is radiation for the early localised case, cytotoxics for the later generalised case. For individual groups of nodes, or deposits in bone, etc, simple techniques delivering 3-4000 rads by single or parallel fields in about three weeks, used to give excellent local results. But nodes in adjacent or other regions sooner or later enlarged, and though successive local treatments were satisfactory for a time, malignancy eventually generalised beyond control. Hence the poor prognosis from this piecemeal approach – though a few cures were achieved. This conservative method has now been abandoned, and replaced by an *aggressive attack on all the lymphatic tissue* in the upper (or lower) half of the body, on one or other side of the diaphragm, in one large single block (Fig. 10.1). If necessary, treatment of one half can be followed by treatment of the other – i.e. *total nodal irradiation* (TNI). It is this new and radical approach that is responsible for the changed outlook, made possible by megavoltage equipment.

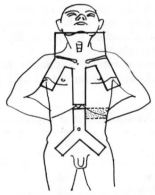

Fig. 10.1 Fields for nodal irradiation, e.g. Hodgkin's. The upper field covers the nodes above the diaphragm ('mantle' technique). The lower field covers the nodes below the diaphragm (inverted Y). Matching posterior fields are used. The upper part of the abdominal fields can be extended on left side to include the spleen or splenic pedicle.

In a Stage I or II case, with nodes of neck, axilla or mediastinum involved, radiation is by the method shown in Fig. 10.1. From its resemblance to a cloak it is known as the *'mantle' technique*. Large anterior and posterior fields cover the whole of the neck, from mastoid processes downwards, plus infraclavicular and pectoro – axillary areas, plus the whole of the mediastinum down to the level of the 12th dorsal vertebra.

The upper border is at the level of the mandible, and the mouth is excluded. It is not usually necessary to include the tonsillar region (Waldeyer's ring) unless there is evidence of involvement. If so, the fields must go up to the base of the skull, front and back. The thoracic section must be carefully shaped on the simulator if available, by means of lead blocks. The mediastinum must be fully included. It is not possible to avoid the apical parts of the lungs, but the rest is shielded.

The tumour dose should be 3500 rads minimum in four weeks.

Treatment below the diaphragm is by large inverted Y fields (Fig. 10.1) covering paraortic and pelvic nodes. If total nodal irradiation is carried out, the second course should follow the first after 4-6 weeks.

The previous lymphogram is invaluable in shaping the outlines of the fields, since the contrast medium is visible on fluoroscopic screen or film. This enables the therapist to use adequate but not excessive margins and so keep the volume dose (and pelvic bone marrow dose) to a minimum. Dosage is of the same order as for the mantle.

In females this technique involves ovarian sterilisation. Some workers have attempted, for younger women, to avoid this by operative removal of at least one ovary from its lateral position in the pelvis and anchoring it in the midline. It would thus receive only scattered radiation, about 100-200 rads, which would have no clinically significant effect (but would carry some risk of genetic damage to future offspring).

With these very large treated volumes − especially the inverted Y − reactions are to be expected, nausea, sore throat, diarrhoea etc, and are managed on the usual lines. Frequent blood counts, including platelets, are essential, and low counts may require suspension of treatment for a few days. The patient should be in hospital if possible, especially for the abdominal course.

For elderly or frail patients, or for treatment of isolated deposits, where aggressive therapy is not suitable, the old-fashioned local methods should be used.

*Cytotoxic chemotherapy.* For Stage IIIB and IV, and for recurrences after radical radiation, chemotherapy is indicated. Formerly, single agents were used, with poor or modest results. Current regimes use multiple agents in combination, and results are outstandingly good. Remissions are nearly always achieved, and patients can be kept going for long years by judiciously spaced and repeated courses. Details are given in Ch. 13.

*Prognosis.* Modern radiotherapy, plus combination chemotherapy, has improved the overall five-year survival from under 40 per cent in the 1940s to over 60 per cent. For stages I and II, 90 per cent is now being achieved, and even 70 per cent for stage III at major centres. Very careful staging and selection of appropriate therapy is essential, to obtain these excellent results, and this is the justification for all the elaborate measures described above. Even in late stages, the results of chemotherapy have been so good that it now seems likely that normal life expectancy is being achieved in some cases. It seems possible that chemotherapy may come to be the treatment of choice even for the early stages.

## Non-Hodgkin's lymphoma

This is a group with a wide range of malignancy, from semi-benign to rapidly aggressive. They may be staged in a way similar to that for Hodgkin's. Management varies according to the histological type and degree of spread. Many of the principles outlined for Hodgkin's disease are applicable, with individual variations. Laparotomy is rarely indicated, unless required for initial diagnosis or removal of involved stomach or bowel.

*Reticulum cell sarcoma.* This is the least radiosensitive and carries the worst prognosis. Node enlargement is the commonest presentation, but there may be involvement of tonsil, bone, bowel, etc.

For Stages IA and IIA, radical radiotherapy should be given us for Hodgkin's. Otherwise chemotherapy and palliative radiotherapy are used.

*Lymphosarcoma.* The radiosensitivity is as good as for Hodgkin's, but the prognosis is not so good. Involvement of stomach or bowel is relatively common and may be the first sign. (Gastric lymphoma is discussed on p. 147).

There may be an associated lymphatic leukaemia, or this may appear terminally. The general lines of management are: radiation for local masses and cytotoxics for generalised disease. Some cases with a solitary focus, e.g. tonsil, are easily curable locally, and may remain permanently free of disease (Fig. 10.2).

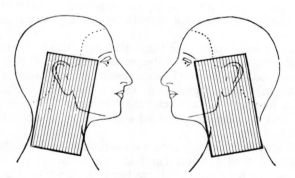

Fig. 10.2. Large-field therapy for reticulosis. Suitable e.g. for lesions confined to tonsil. Two fields, 25 × 15 cm, at 250 kV or 4 MV, to include whole of pharynx and adjacent lymph-node areas. *(Paterson, Treatment of Malignant Disease, 2nd edition, Arnold)*

*Follicular lymphoma:* This is the least aggressive of the group, and the most radiosensitive. It carries the best prognosis of all. There are often spontaneous remissions. Treatment can afford to be on non-aggressive lines. Doses of 3000 rads in three weeks are adequate for local control.

## Mycosis fungoides

This is a neoplasm of the reticular tissue of the skin, with some characteristic features. It runs a very chronic course, via a pre-mycotic phase of dermatitis for many years. There are itching erythematous patches, which later become thickened to form plaques, and finally fungating tumours, often likened to tomatoes. There may be terminal visceral involvement, of liver, etc.

Individual lesions are very radiosensitive, and palliation can be given, often for years, by superficial radiation. Doses of a few hundred rads usually suffice. Superficial electron therapy is also useful, either to small patches or to large areas — even the whole trunk or body — from linear accelerators, betatrons or iridium units. In the later stages, cytotoxics may help, combined with steroids.

*Burkitt's lymphoma* is another special member of the lympho-reticular group. (It is described on p. 233).

## Leukaemia

Leukaemia is a group of diseases characterised by cancerous proliferation of leukopoietic (white cell forming) tissue throughout the body, chiefly bone marrow and lymphoid tissue. The incidence is everywhere increasing and has more than doubled in the past 25 years. The cause is unknown, but there is an undoubted relation to exposure to ionising radiation:

a. Survivors of the atom bomb explosions at Hiroshima and Nagasaki showed a twenty-fold increase as compared with normals.

b. Patients treated by X-rays for ankylosing spondylitis have a six-fold incidence (see p. 248).

c. Doctors, especially radiologists, are at greater risk than the general population.

An infective virus has been found to produce leukaemia experimentally in some animals, but there is no evidence of an infective origin in humans.

*Pathology.* White blood cells are of several types, and any type may undergo the malignant change, so that we can classify the varieties of leukaemia according to the particular cell type. The normal process of transformation of primitive stem cells into mature adult cells is somehow disturbed and arrested, so that these primitive cells accumulate in the marrow and enter the circulation in large numbers, to give the typical peripheral blood picture. The marrow becomes filled with leukaemic cells which crowd out other components — red cells (with resultant anaemia) and platelets (with resultant impaired blood clotting and tendency to haemorrhage).

Resistance to infection is lowered because of the immaturity of the white cells. The end comes with failure of normal marrow function — severe anaemia and usually terminal infection or haemorrhage.

The chief varieties are (a) *lymphatic*; (b) *myeloid* or *granulocytic* leukaemia – arising from the lymphocytic series or the polymorphonuclear leucocytes. Rarer types are the monocytic and eosinophil leukaemias.

Leukaemia is also subdivided into (a) *acute* and (b) *chronic* types, according to the rapidity of the clinical course, but the malignant process is essentially similar apart from the time factor.

*Acute leukaemia* may be lymphatic, myeloid or other type, but the clinical picture is similar in all. It may occur at any age, but is most common in childhood (see p. 236). The onset is usually sudden, with fever, sore throat and bleeding from mouth or elsewhere. Typically there is a total white cell count of 20 000-50 000 per cubic mm, of which about 90 per cent are very immature or blast cells (lymphoblasts, myeloblasts, etc.). The diagnosis is obvious on the blood film, and is confirmed on examination of bone marrow, obtained from sternum or iliac crest, which shows heavy infiltration with blast cells. Often the cells are so primitive that it is impossible to say whether they are of lymphoid or myeloid type.

Some cases are at first aleukaemic, i.e. there is no excess of leucocytes in peripheral blood, but the marrow shows typical appearances.

*Chronic leukaemia* is of two main types – lymphatic or myeloid (granulocytic). The cells are more mature than in acute cases, and the clinical course is much more prolonged, with periods of spontaneous remission, before the fatal outcome. Diagnosis rests on the cells in peripheral blood and marrow.

a. *Chronic myeloid leukaemia* occurs mainly in early adult life and middle age. The typical picture is of progressive tiredness due to anaemia, with gross splenic enlargement which may cause a dragging sensation in the abdomen. The spleen may reach a huge size and appear to fill most of the abdomen. Lymph nodes are not usually enlarged. Occasionally there is leukaemic infiltration of the skin. The blood count shows a total white count between 100 000 and 500 000, of which 50 to 70 per cent are polymorphs and 10-20 per cent myelocytes (precursors of the polymorphs). There is always some degree of anaemia.

b. *Chronic lymphatic leukaemia* is usually seen in men of late middle age. The onset is insidious, with tiredness from anaemia. Enlargement of spleen, liver, lymphnodes of neck, axillae and elsewhere, is found. The spleen does not reach the huge size of the chronic myeloid variety. The blood shows a total white count up to 100 000, of which 80 to 90 per cent are small lymphocytes, and associated anaemia. Leukaemic infiltration of skin, bone etc., may occur.

### Treatment

A. *Acute leukaemia* is treated mainly by *cytotoxic chemotherapy* – see Ch. 13. This has given remarkable and revolutionary results in the last decade, and the prognosis has been radically improved.

*Radiation* however has an essential supplementary role, to treat the central nervous system (CNS), which is usually involved by leukaemic deposits on the meninges. These cells are not effectively reached by the drugs given by mouth or intravenous injection, since they do not cross the 'blood-brain barrier'. If they are not specially dealt with, they will cause relapses, with headache, vomiting etc. All patients should therefore be given 'prophylactic' therapy, early in the period of remission, 6 to 8 weeks after diagnosis. Its great value has been proved by experience.

There are two techniques: (a) irradiation of the entire cranio-spinal axis; (b) irradiation of the cranium combined with intrathecal injection of a cytotoxic drug. In the first method, radiation is applied in the same manner as for medulloblastoma (see p. 152) giving 2400 rads by megavoltage in three weeks but in this case the posterior part of the orbit should be included. For children under two years, use 2000 rads; under one year, 1500. In the other method, a similar dose is given to cranium only, and the rest of the CNS treated by intrathecal Methotrexate five doses given twice weekly. Temporary alopecia is usual with either method, and wigs should be ordered beforehand, at least for the girls.

Local radiation is also valuable for relief of bone or joint pain. Single doses of 200-300 rads suffice.

*Supportive therapy*, important in all types and phases of leukaemia, especially the acute, can be crucial, e.g. blood transfusion for severe anaemia, antibiotics for infection. Fluid intake must be kept high, to assist the kidneys to eliminate the breakdown products of destroyed leukaemic cells.

*Immunotherapy* is also proving helpful. The body's defence system can be stimulated by injections of vaccine, e.g. B.C.G., given between the courses of chemotherapy.

*Results* in the acute myeloid type (AML) are definitely inferior to those of lymphatic (ALL). But remission rates of over 50 per cent can now be achieved in adults by intensive chemotherapy. Early relapse, however, is the rule, and the prognosis still remains extremely poor, in contrast to childhood (p. 237).

*B. Chronic leukaemia* is also now treated mainly by drugs, notably Busulphan (see p. 224). Radiation used to be the mainstay of treatment, and still has its uses. The aim of treatment is to relieve symptoms and maintain the quality of life. No treatment is needed if the general condition is satisfactory and white cell count and haemoglobin levels reasonable. The best indicator for treatment is a fall in haemoglobin, which usually goes along with a rise in the white count. Treatment may also be required if an enlarged spleen causes symptoms; or node masses may be troublesome, even if only psychologically. Regular blood counts are essential, and should be charted graphically, so that the rate as well as the extent of change can be followed. A total white count of 10-15 000 is aimed at, and as the total falls the haemoglobin level usually rises, with improvement of symptoms. Too much attention should not be paid to the actual white total, and it is not essential to bring it down to these levels; some patients feel better with a higher count. The haemoglobin level is the more important indicator. Care must be taken not to overshoot the mark by excessive treatment which may inhibit the marrow so effectively as to lower the white count to dangerously low levels and expose the patient to devastating infection.

*Radiation* may be used for: (a) local treatment of the spleen, especially in the granulocytic type; (b) local treatment of lymphnode masses, (c) local deposits in bone, skin or elsewhere. (d) total body irradiation.

a. Radiation to the spleen used to be the standard form of therapy and is usually quite effective in lowering the white count. It is also useful for decreasing the mass of an uncomfortably large spleen or controlling pain from perisplenitis (irritation from inflammatory involvement of the capsule of the spleen). To lower the white count it is not necessary to irradiate the whole of the spleen. Simple direct anterior or lateral fields, e.g. 15 × 10 cm are adequate. Treatment should be gradual, beginning with 25 rads incident and increasing by 25 a day to about 150 to 200. Daily blood counts are made, and the course continues till the level is judged low enough. The number of doses will depend on the rapidity of the response, bearing in mind that the drop will continue for several days after the last dose. Although the disease is widespread, satisfactory control for a long time is generally possible by splenic irradiation alone. The spleen is one of the chief sites of production of the abnormal white cells, but the effects of splenic irradiation are not confined to the spleen – there is also a distant effect on bone marrow, etc. in a way not understood. Courses of radiation to the spleen can be repeated, but eventually resistance develops, just as it does to any form of therapy in leukaemia. Splenic irradiation is seldom indicated in lymphatic leukaemia.

b. & c. For node masses or local deposits, low doses of 500 to 1000 rads are usually adequate. Node irradiation is more often indicated in the lymphatic type, and the white count usually falls at the same time as a result.

d. Total body radiation was used mainly for the granulocytic type. Either radio-phosphorus (P-32) was given (orally or intravenously) or external radiation encompassing the whole body at increased FSD. These methods have in most centres been superseded by multi-drug regimes, but may still be of value on occasion.

Eventually the time comes when therapy no longer avails, and marrow failure sets in. Symptomatic and supportive therapy alone are then indicated – transfusion, antibiotics, sedatives etc.

*Prognosis.* In acute leukaemia the picture has recently changed dramatically, because of cytotoxics. Life expectation used to be a matter of months and early death inevitable. The greatest change has been in acute lymphoblastic leukaemia, which is the typical form in childhood. With modern intensive therapy, i.e. multi-drug regimes plus CNS radiation, patients are surviving ten years and more. We are now beginning to talk of 'cure', though the treatment is so recent that it will be many years before we can be sure. It is reasonable to believe that *at least 25 per cent can now be permanently controlled.* This is one of the most spectacular 'breakthroughs' of modern medicine.

In chronic leukaemia the picture is different, and there have been no major advances. Chronic lymphatic leukaemia is sometimes almost benign, with a slow course over 10 to 20 years and very little in the way of symptoms. But average survival in chronic types is only 2 to 4 years, and current treatment probably has little effect on length of life, though it can improve the quality.

## Polycythaemia

(Polycythaemia Rubra Vera, Primary Polycythaemia).

This is an uncommon disease of bone marrow, mostly in middle aged males. There is hyperplasia of all constituents – erythroblastic, leucoblastic, megakaryocytic – i.e. the precursors of red and white cells and platelets, which are all increased in the peripheral blood. The clinical picture is dominated by the greatly increased number of red cells in the peripheral circulation (hence the name), but there may eventually be complete marrow exhaustion (aplastic anaemia), or the erythroblastic tissue may be exhausted first and the leucoblastic proliferation continue, leading to leukaemia.

*Clinical features.* The patient complains of headache, dizziness and tiredness, and has a cyanosed plethoric appearance. The spleen is palpably enlarged. The increase in the red cell volume decreases the fluidity of the blood, i.e. there is increased viscosity leading to thromboses (in brain, limbs, etc.) and haemorrhages.

The red cell count may be up to 10 million or more, with equivalent increase in haemoglobin. The red cell volume is increased; this is the haematocrit or packed cell volume, i.e. the volume occupied by the red cells in 100 ml of centrifuged blood, normally about 45 per cent.

Other causes of polycythaemia must be excluded before making the diagnosis. *Secondary polycythaemia* can occur from the stimulus of anoxia (decreased oxygen caused by deficient oxygenation of the blood) at high attitudes, in congenital heart disease and in certain lung diseases. It may also be found associated with renal lesions, especially cancer of the kidney. The bone marrow picture is also helpful in distinguishing the various types.

*Treatment.* The aim is to produce a prolonged reduction of the red cell volume to a fairly normal level. This may be done by: (a) venesection; (b) chemotherapy or (c) radiation.

Venesection (vein puncture) reduces blood volume rapidly and so gives quick symptomatic relief. It may be technically difficult because the high viscosity makes the blood flow very sluggishly. The effects is very temporary, since it does nothing to remove the cause in the marrow. It may be useful, e.g. before an operation, to decrease the danger of thrombosis.

Cytotoxic chemotherapy (usually busulphan) can be given in short courses, repeated as necessary. Prolonged treatment is needed, with close supervision and frequent blood counts. Most centres have given it up in favour of radiation.

Radiation used to be given either to the spleen, by trunk baths or whole body baths. These have now been almost entirely superseded by *radioactive phosphorus* (P-32) which is much easier and more convenient. Dosage is empirical, usually 4 to 7 millicuries intravenously, according to the patient's weight and the severity of the case. It can also be given orally, 8 to 12 mc to allow for incomplete absorption from the bowel. The patient need not be in hospital, since the radioactivity excreted in urine, etc. is not of a dangerous order. The red cell count begins to fall in 6 to 8 weeks, and a repeat dose is not given for at least three months. A decision to re-treat is based on clinical and haematological findings and the required dose is modified in the light of these.

About 85 per cent achieve excellent remission, and most of them need only a single injection for this. The very few who prove resistant are treated by chemotherapy or venesection every month or so. The length of remission varies considerably, averaging about two years.

One possible disadvantage of P-32 is that it may cause late leukaemia, but this can occur in any event. P-32 probably does raise the incidence slightly, but on balance the risk is quite acceptable, and it is the treatment of choice in almost all cases.

*Prognosis.* Without treatment, the average survival is about five years, but modern therapy has more than doubled this. The end comes with marrow failure, leukaemia, thrombosis, haemorrhage or heart failure.

**Myelomatosis** (Multiple Myeloma)

This is a disease of bone marrow, occurring in late middle age.

*Pathology.* The cell concerned is the plasma cell, which is believed to arise from the primitive reticulum cells of the marrow. Neoplastic proliferation leads to marrow destruction, failure, and also to local destruction of bone, so that this lesion is often classified with bone tumours.

A remarkable feature is that the plasma cells produce abnormal proteins, which appear in the blood and can easily be detected. Abnormal proteins may also be found in the urine (Bence-Jones protein). Renal failure may occur from plugging of renal tubules with precipitated protein.

*Clinical features.* The most common symptom is bone pain, e.g. from a vertebra or rib. Radiographs may show generalised bone rarefaction (osteoporosis) or very characteristic punched-out osteolytic lesions, especially in skull, ribs and vertebrae. Pathological fractures are common, or collapse of vertebrae with serious neurological complications, including paraplegia from compression of spinal cord.

Diagnosis is confirmed by examination of bone marrow, which reveals the typical plasma cells.

*Treatment* is unsatisfactory. Localised bone pain can usually be relieved by external radiation, e.g. 3000 rads incident over the affected part of the spine, by DXR or cobalt beam, in two weeks. Generalised radiation with P-32 (dosage and intervals as for polycythaemia – see above) may be helpful in widespread involvement.

Chemotherapy is also widely used, and can give useful results. The chief drugs are: melphalan, cyclophosphamide and steroids.

Supportive therapy is important, especially blood transfusion for anaemia. Pathological fracture may need operation and pinning (see p. 170).

*Prognosis* is very variable, but most die within 2 to 3 years. Intensive drug therapy may add another year or so to life expectation in those who respond.

*Solitary myeloma (Plasmacytoma) of bone.* Myeloma confined to a single bone is unusual. When it does occur it can be successfully treated by local radiation: 3500-4000 rads in 3 to 4 weeks. Most cases however, develop multiple lesions eventually, though it may not be till several years later.

### Extramedullary plasmacytoma

Plasma cell tumours may appear in organs other than bone marrow, and are sometimes benign, but may be the first manifestation of multiple myeloma. The commonest sites are in the upper air passages e.g. larynx.

### Ewing's tumour

This is an uncommon but characteristic tumour in bone, usually in a child or young adult. Its pathological nature is disputed, but it is probably a reticulum cell sarcoma of bone marrow, and not a primary bone tumour. Some apparent cases have proved to be secondary to a neuroblastoma discovered at post-mortem examination. It arises usually in the shaft of a long bone, causing pain. It may be mistaken at first for an inflammatory bone lesion (osteomyelitis). Radiography shows a typical appearance; central erosion with surrounding subperiosteal new-- bone, giving an 'onion skin' picture. Early and wide spread is usual, especially to other bones and lungs. Secondaries in regional nodes occur less commonly.

Diagnosis must be confirmed by surgical biopsy.

*Treatment.* The tumour is highly radiosensitive, and local control is obtainable, but metastasis is very much the rule and hardly any cases survive five years. Amputation is scarcely ever justified, since external radiation usually achieves local control. The whole bone (not just the apparently affected part of the bone) should receive about 5000 rads in 4 to 5 weeks, which secures pain relief and local healing. Similar treatment may be given to metastases in other bones. Even lung deposits can be successfully treated with doses of 2000 to 3000 rads.

*Cytotoxic drugs* are now improving the outlook. The optimum regime is intensive radiation to heal the local lesion, with concurrent chemotherapy to deal with microscopic secondary deposits. Multiple agents should be used in combination – actinomycin – D, adriamycin, vincristine and cyclophosphamide – preferably all four together. Chemotherapy is continued for at least two years, with treatment – free intervals.

*Prognosis*. Surgery and/or radiation give cure rates under 10 per cent. Intensive chemotherapy is now achieving much improved survival.

# 11. Radioactive Isotopes in Therapy

*The Worldly Hope men set their Hearts upon*
*Turns Ashes — or it prospers; and anon,*
*Like Snow upon the Desert's dusty Face*
*Lighting a little Hour or two — is gone.*
                    Edward Fitzgerald (Omar Khayyam)

The properties, production, etc. of radioactive isotopes, both natural and artificial, are described in Chapter 4 and Table 11.1, which include a brief account of their diagnostic use as tracers and as substitutes for radium in therapy in the form of sealed sources.

In this chapter we shall describe a few more sealed sources, but concentrate mainly on the uses of *unsealed (liquid) sources* in radiotherapy departments and wards. The chief of these are:

1. Iodine                  3. Gold
2. Phosphorus              4. Yttrium

The following are *sealed sources:*

5. Strontium               6. Iridium

Strontium is also used as an unsealed source in tracer studies (p. 52).

*Internal administration* to the patient, by mouth or injection, results as a rule in active material entering the bloodstream and so being distributed widely throughout the body, and passing out of the therapist's control. This is virtually a new field of radiotherapy, where a host of new problems arise.

## General problems

*Metabolism and tissue selectivity.*

A radioactive element behaves chemically exactly like its inactive stable relative, enters into the same chemical reactions and goes through the same metabolic processes. Different organs will have different affinities for different elements, and this is of fundamental importance in determining their final distribution, and both their usefulness and their danger.

*The best example — indeed the only really good example — of highly selective absorption by an organ is the take-up of radioactive iodine by the thyroid gland.*

In the early days, when artificial radioactivity became practicable — about 1940 — it seemed that the 'magic bullet' to destroy cancer cells was just around the corner. But these high hopes have been sadly disappointed, and the cancericidal radioactive drug remains still a dream.

*Protection.* Special problems obviously arise in the handling of radioactive material, in measuring it, preparing it for the patient, avoiding contamination in laboratory and ward, protecting nursing, medical and other staff, and disposing of waste products of the patient. These are dealt with in Chapter 7.

*Late effects.* In the reproductive years, the *genetic effects* on ovary and testis must be considered (p. 94). So must the possibility of *late carcinogenesis* in tissues where isotopes are concentrated, e.g. leukaemia in bone marrow, cancer in the thyroid — compare the devastating effects in

Table 11.1 Radioactive isotopes used in therapy

| Element | Symbol | Main radiations | Half-life | Main uses |
|---------|--------|-----------------|-----------|-----------|
| Radium | Ra-226 | Beta Gamma | 1600 years | Needles and tubes, for interstitial implantation, intra-cavitary insertion and surface application. |
| Cobalt | Co-60 | Gamma | 5.3 years | Telecobalt units. Radium substitute, as needles or tubes |
| Caesium | Cs-137 | Gamma | 30 years | Telecaesium units. Radium substitute, as needles or tubes. |
| Strontium | Sr-90 | Beta | 28 years | Surface treatment, especially in ophthalmology |
| Iridium | Ir-192 | Gamma | 74 days | Beam unit; also radium substitute, flexible wire for implantation (e.g. bladder) |
| Iodine | I-131 | Beta Gamma | 8 days | Systemic (oral) for hyperthyroidism, thyroid cancer and thyroid ablation. |
| Gold | Au-198 | Beta Gamma | 2.7 days | As grains, for interstitial implantation. In solution, for instillation into serous cavities. |
| Yttrium | Y-90 | Beta | 2.5 days | In solution, for instillation into serous cavities. As solid rod, for interstitial pituitary ablation. |
| Phosphorus | P-32 | Beta | 14.3 days | Systemic (I.V. – also oral) especially for polycythaemia. In solution, for instillation into serous cavities. |

the watch dial painters (p. 14). In treatment of cancer, these risks are acceptable, but caution is indicated in non-malignant disorders such as thyrotoxicosis.

## Radioactive iodine and the thyroid gland

Radioactive iodine is a valuable tool in the treatment of two disorders of the thyroid gland: (a) *Thyrotoxicosis* (hyperthyroidism), (b) *Cancer*.

The thyroid gland synthesizes the hormone thyroxine (T4), which is essential for the maintenance of normal metabolism, utilising iodine from the diet. As with other endocrine function, the activity of the thyroid is controlled by the pituitary through the *thyroid stimulating hormone TSH*. By substituting radioactive iodine, this unique affinity for the chemical provides a useful method of producing a high dose of radiation within a very small volume of tissue.

There are several radioactive isotopes of iodine, of which the most important is $^{131}$I. Its half-life is eight days and it emits mainly beta rays, but also a proportion of gamma rays. The betas are all absorbed within a few millimetres of tissue, but the gammas are far more penetrating and even from a small quantity of $^{131}$I, enough of them emerge from the thyroid and through the skin surface to allow detection and measurement by an external counter or scanner (p. 53-4).

When given to a patient, it is *metabolised exactly like ordinary iodine,* taken up by the thyroid and used for the synthesis of hormone.

## Thyrotoxicosis

This is a clinical state associated with raised levels of circulating thyroxine (T4) and sometimes other thyroid hormones. As a result there is an increase in the body metabolism manifested by agitation, palpitations, profuse sweating and weight loss. The disease affects females more commonly than males and usually in the 40-60 age group. There is sometimes a significant enlargement of the thyroid gland. Occasionally when a large gland extends behind the sternum (retrosternal extension) there may be evidence of obstruction of the trachea.

*The high iodine affinity provides methods of diagnosis as well as treatment.*

## Investigation of thyroid function

The important tests of the thyroid function are those associated with the uptake of radioactive iodine ( $^{131}$I, $^{132}$I) or other isotopes (Technetium). These may provide a measure of the physiological activity of the gland (tracer techniques) or provide a measure of size and position (imaging or scanning). Both of these tests require sophisticated apparatus and are *in vivo* (i.e. performed on the patient) but recent tests – which are biochemical – can be performed in the laboratory (*in vitro*) on samples of blood. In most cases it is necessary to perform a large spectrum of tests which provide the information from which the diagnosis is made.

### The tracer investigation

This has become a routine procedure, and is particularly useful in helping to separate doubtful cases from, e.g. anxiety neurosis. It is usually done on an out-patient basis.

The patient attends in the isotope laboratory before breakfast and takes a very small dose of $^{131}$I (15 µ Ci – see p. 52) diluted in water and drunk through a straw. He may return home for breakfast and report back four hours later. He then lies on a couch, and a counter above the neck measures the radiation emittted from the gland (Fig. 11.1). This gives a measure of the amount of $^{131}$I which has been absorbed by the cells of the thyroid from the test drink, following its passage from the gut into the bloodstream. The count is repeated at 48 hours, when a blood sample is also taken; and the $^{131}$I content of the blood proteins is estimated. In some cases, e.g. suspected myxoedema, the urinary content of $^{131}$I is also measured.

### Interpretation of the tracer test.

The functioning of the normal and the hyperactive gland is shown in Fig. 11.3.

a. *Gland.* Normally the measured radioactivity rises gently to a plateau, reached soon after 24 hours, but the toxic gland removes iodine from the blood at such a rapid rate that the $^{131}$I curve rises to a sharp peak in a few hours and then falls. Thus the measured 4-hour uptake will distinguish most thyrotoxic cases quite definitely.

b. *Plasma.* Normally the blood is cleared of iodine gradually, and at 48 hours very little is left, but in the toxic cases there is a secondary rise due to secretion of newly formed hormone, incorporating some of the $^{131}$I. The 48 hour figures give almost conclusive evidence in most cases.

c. *Urine.* Most of the $^{131}$I not absorbed by the thyroid is excreted in the urine and the urinary concentration of $^{131}$I is much lower in the toxic case, since the rapidity of uptake by the thyroid leaves much less in the bloodstream to be excreted. Assays of urine are not necessary in most thyrotoxic cases and are not routinely done, but may be of value in assessment of myxoedema where a sluggish thyroid takes up less iodine than normal, leaving more for urinary excretion.

### The thyroid scan

An image of the gland may be obtained by giving the patient a small quantity of radioactive iodine or technetium (see above) and using a special detector.

The *rectilinear scanner* will 'look' at the activity within the gland in automated 1cm steps and produce a composite colour picture of the size and shape of the gland with areas of high (red) and low (blue) activity clearly defined (See Fig. 11.2).

The gamma camera is a sophisticated measuring device which looks at the whole of the gland at the same instant and produces an image which can be recorded on a photographic plate.

Variation in shape and activity are easily detected and the test is invaluable in revealing retrosternal goitre and particularly in investigation of thyroid cancer.

Other useful tests of thyroid function includes:

a. Measurement of circulating thyroxine by chemical means (as distinct from the radioactive test).

Normal range 4-12 μ g/100 ml.

b. Measurement of TSH – normal range up to 4 mu/l. The level is low in thyrotoxicosis.

c. T3 Resin uptake – which determines the amount of free T.B.G. (= Thyroid Binding Globulin).

## The treatment of thyrotoxicosis

A small proportion of patients with thyrotoxicosis will improve spontaneously but active treatment is required in most patients. Essentially treatment is concerned with the reduction of circulating thyroxine, either by the partial destruction of the gland or by interrupting the synthesis of the hormone.

Destructive therapy may be achieved either by surgery (removal of most of the thyroid gland) or by using the special radioactive iodine in carefully measured doses. Both methods have a place in the management of hyperthyroidism but radioactive iodine therapy has the advantage of being relatively simple and devoid of serious side effects and complications. Medical control is achieved by the use of a variety of drugs, such as Carbimazole (10 mg q.d.s. initially, reducing to 5-15 mg daily) and Propylthiouracil (100 mg q.d.s.). Drug therapy may be accompanied by serious side effects but is often used as a preliminary method of treatment. It may be especially important where surgery or $^{131}$I cannot be used because of other medical conditions, poor general condition or pregnancy.

## Radioactive iodine therapy

The technique is simple. A dose calculated from the size of the gland and the uptake of radioactive iodine (in the tracer test) is given to the patient under the same conditions as for the diagnostic test. Unless the patient is ill, this can be arranged on an out-patient basis – although the patient should stay at the hospital for a few hours until the possibility of vomiting and other side effects has subsided. The size of the therapeutic drink is of the order of 2-8 m Ci which is usually sufficiently low to avoid the need for special precautions to prevent contamination and ensure the safety of staff. If the disease is not controlled by a single treatment, then more doses may be necessary having allowed 2-3 months to elapse after each dose in order to assess the full effect.

The drawback of this treatment is the progressive effect of the irradiation, which leads to increasing atrophy of the gland with a slow decrease in the amount of circulating thyroxine, which produces hypothyroidism – the clinical syndrome of myxoedema.

This treatment is usually restricted to patients over 40, because of the theoretical risk of inducing leukaemia or thyroid cancer – though this has never occurred after more than 20 years experience. There is also the possibility of gene mutations in the reproductive cells of ovary and testis.

If treatment is carried out on the ward, isolation is not necessary nor is a separate toilet usually required. If urine needs to be collected, most patients can do this themselves and put the urine in a special labelled collecting bottle kept in the toilet. If the patient is confined to bed, the physicists will usually advise on the precautions which should be observed.

## Malignancy in the thyroid

Cancer of the thyroid is a rare disease, only twelve new patients occurring each year in a million population. However, the disease tends to be commoner in the goitregenic areas, e.g. Derbyshire, Switzerland, and because of especial interests these patients tend to be seen in units specialising in the treatment of thyroid disorders. The common thyroid cancer is the adenocarcinoma and there is a distinct and interesting age incidence of the two main types (a) well-differentiated and (b) anaplastic.

*The well differentiated tumour,* which histologically may be indistinguishable from normal thyroid tissue and often functions as normal thyroid tissue, occurs in the younger age group 10 to 50 years. It is usually relatively slow growing and has a good prognosis. In the older age group (60 to 90) the tumour is usually the rapidly growing *anaplastic tumour,* which is physiologically inert, widely metastasising and unfortunately usually rapidly fatal. This cancer is best dealt with by X-ray therapy, although surgery is sometimes required to relieve troublesome pressure effects.

In the well differentiated tumour there is no place for external irradiation but in a small number of cases (about 5 per cent) radioactive iodine may have an important part to play.

However, the *main treatment* in this group of patients, which form about one third of all patients with malignant thyroid growths, is *surgical removal of the whole (total thyroidectomy) or part of the gland (usually lobectomy).* Because of the way in which some of these cancers spread, it is advisable to remove any enlarged nodes in the neck as well. Histological examination of the tissue removed at operation will give some indication of the physiological activity of a tumour, but generally *the tumour will only manifest its ability to utilize iodine after the normal thyroid has been removed.* The logical approach to treatment is, therefore:

a. Destruction of all normal thyroid tissue.
b. Assessment of volume and site of functioning thyroid tissue.
c. Destruction of functioning thyroid tissue.

The treatment may extend over a long period of time and the first step in patients with operable tumours is to remove as much normal thyroid as possible by total thyroidectomy. Radioactive iodine is then given to destroy any tissue that remains. The amount of [131]I is much larger than that needed in the treatment of hyperthyroidism and special precaution has to be taken to avoid contamination (see below). If the cancer is inoperable, treatment commences with several large amounts of [131]I over a period of 6-12 weeks.

Destructive amounts of [131]I of this order are normally referred to as *ablation doses* and result in a *complete cessation of thyroid function and produce hypothyroidism*. For the patient this is an unpleasant, unhappy state resulting in sluggishness, coldness and rapid weight increase, but before reversing the condition by giving thyroxine, it is important to scan and assess the amount of functioning tissue, if any. The scan not only examines the neck areas but also the lungs and skeleton − possible sites for metastases.

If function cannot be demonstrated − the hypothyroidism is reversed by giving thyroxine in tablet form 0.3 mg daily (there is no need for this dose to be divided, e.g. 0.1 mg t.d.s.). As well as its importance as a replacement for normal thyroid, however, this drug may suppress tumour recurrence (see below). Where there is still functioning thyroid tissue, further drinks of [131]I are given until it has been completely destroyed.

The progress of the disease is monitored by performing scans at frequent intervals and giving further drinks of [131]I as and when required. These should be performed 3 or 6 monthly in the first year after diagnosis, but once the disease is under control the need for such investigation becomes less important, but the patient should be under surveillance preferably at a special clinic.

It is impossible to obtain a meaningful scan whilst the patient is taking large doses of thyroxine by mouth and in order to produce optimum conditions which will allow any residual thyroid tissue to function, thyroxine (T4) needs to be discontinued at least four weeks before the scan is performed. The misery of hypothyroidism may be alleviated by substituting a short acting thyroid hormone, tri-iodothyronine (T3) (20 $\mu$g 8 hourly) for thyroxine (T4) a month before the scan is required and continuing T3 up to a week before the test is performed. In circumstances where scans are required at frequent intervals, it is obviously advisable to use Tri-iodothyronine (T3) until the disease is under control but this drug should not be used for long periods of time.

The ablation and therapy drinks of [131]I are seldom accompanied by side effects and the patient needs to be hospitalised only because of the precautions associated with contamination and can usually be discharged after 2-3 days. The full effects of radioactive iodine therapy may not be apparent for several months, so that the total duration of treatment may be prolonged. Occasionally where many large amounts of radioactive iodine have been given, there are problems with bone marrow depression.

### Nursing problems associated with $^{131}$I therapy

All ablation and therapy doses of $^{131}$I are large (e.g. 100 ml) because of the small amount that is concentrated in functioning thyroid tissue; most of the radioactivity is excreted, mainly by the urine, very rapidly and any problems associated with radioactive safety usually occur within the first 48 hours after the dose. During this period, however, strict precautions are observed and because of particular problems it is wise always to ask for the guidance of the isotope physicists in each particular case.

The therapeutic drink is given in the isotope laboratory, and the patient should be nursed in a separate side-ward and preferably use a separate toilet. Full precautions must be observed, in accordance with the Local Rules — see section on unsealed sources, pp. 105-6. The chief points to observe are: rubber gloves and aprons for all nursing procedures; separate crockery and washing; bed linen put in plastic bags for monitoring in isotope laboratory; separate bed-pan and bottles. In a large hospital, the urine may be disposed of in the ordinary way and will be diluted to a harmless level in the main drain. In a small hospital, it may be necessary to put all urine on collection into a special container with lead protection; this is removed to a remote cellar until after a week or so the radioactivity falls to a safe level and it can then be disposed of down the drain. The radioactivity of the urine may need to be measured by the physics department, but assay of faeces is very rarely indicated. The nurse should check with the physicist exactly what specimens are required.

In the event of *contamination* (overturned bottle, vomit, etc.) the drill described on p. 106 should be followed. The Local Rules will give guidance on local variations and facilities.

Visitors should be limited as far as possible for a few days after these large doses; they should stay only a short time and sit at a distance. Nurses themselves should be as expeditious as reasonably possible in the room. Waste food should be put in plastic bags for routine monitoring. The meaning and importance of the isolation and precautions should be explained to the patient (and his visitors).

### Hormone suppression therapy

The value of this treatment has not been proved and because of the rarity of thyroid malignancy, it has been difficult to assess. Theoretically it is reasonable to assume that well-differentiated tumours may be stimulated by the thyroid stimulating hormone (TSH) from the pituitary and that, if a primary tumour has been removed, residual tumour and metastases may enlarge because of TSH influence. *The secretion of TSH may be reduced by giving large amounts of exogenous thyroxine by mouth.*

In spite of its doubtful value, this treatment has no side effects and is necessary in the patient in order to reverse the hypothyroidism produced

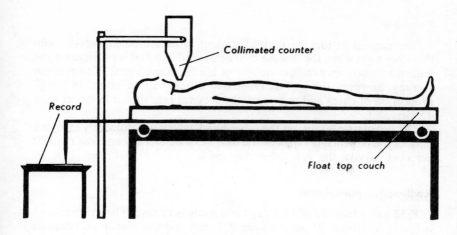

Fig. 11.1 Thyroid scanning. Patient on movable couch under counter (*Paterson, 'Treatment of Malignant Disease', 2nd edition, Arnold*)

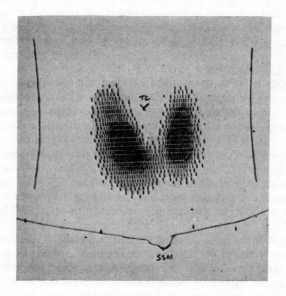

Fig. 11.2. A thyroid scintiscan. In a colour picture the darker central area would be red, the outer area blue.

by thyroid ablation. The majority of patients with well differentiated thyroid cancers receive thyroxine as an adjunct to the definitive treatment.

## Prognosis

The natural history of thyroid tumour is measured in decades and therefore even when the disease cannot be eradicated, it is possible for the patient to enjoy an excellent quality of life for many years. With modern therapy, however, the well differentiated cancer can be 'cured' in a high proportion of cases and at 5 years the survival rate should be better than 75 per cent.

The anaplastic lesion, on the other hand, which unfortunately form the bulk of the patients, is rapidly fatal in spite of all therapy and less than 10 per cent survive the year after diagnosis.

## Radioactive phosphorus

P-32 has a half-life of 14.3 days and emits beta-rays. Their penetration is low − less than 50 per cent reach 1 mm and the maximum range in tissue is only a few millimetres. For therapy, it is prepared usually as a simple salt (sodium phosphate) in solution.

*Biological properties.* Phosphorus is an essential constituent of all cells, especially of nuclei, and is therefore taken up to a greater extent in rapidly dividing cells than in normal cells. It will thus tend to accumulate more in neoplastic tissue and in those normal tissues where growth ordinarily occurs at a relatively fast tempo, such as the blood-forming cells of bone marrow; here the uptake will be even higher in malignant marrow conditions (leukaemia etc.).

*Therapeutic uses.* P-32 is used in two distinct ways:

1. Internally, by ingestion or injection − *via metabolic pathways* after incorporation into cells (like I-131). This is its most important use.

2. Externally − for *surface* beta therapy on internal or external surfaces.

*Internal therapy.* It is best given by intravenous injection with a lead--protected syringe in the isotope laboratory. It can also be given by mouth, though only about three-quarters will be absorbed and the rest lost in the faeces. To secure maximal absorption, the stomach should be empty after a 12-hr fast and the next meal not taken until 3 hr after the dose.

Although P-32 tends to be concentrated in cancer tissue, the degree of concentration is not high enough to be of much practical value − i.e. a substantial dose to a tumour involves unacceptably high dosage to the rest of the body, especially bone marrow, comparable to a total body bath of X-rays. This contrasts unfavourably with the very highly differential absorption of I-131 by the thyroid gland.

The most useful results have been in the reticuloses, above all in polycythaemia (p. 185) where P-32 has now largely replaced other methods.

*P-32 in polycythaemia.* A typical dose is 5 mCi intravenously, or 8

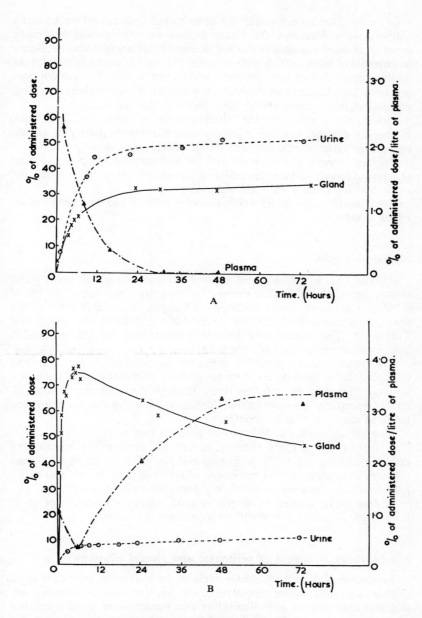

Fig. 11.3 A and B Curves showing results of tracer investigations using $^{131}$I, in typical cases; (a) normal; (b) thyrotoxic.

mCi orally. The red cell count will begin to fall in about 10 weeks and a single dose will restore the blood picture to near normal for many months, or even one or more years. Repeat doses are given as necessary at intervals of not less than three months. The advantages and drawbacks of this simple line of therapy are discussed on p. 186. The patient need not be in hospital, and with the small amounts of radioactivity involved, no special precautions about urine disposal etc. are necessary.

*Other reticuloses.* Similar treatment is possible in leukaemia, Hodgkin's disease, multiple myeloma etc., but has no particular advantages over other treatments and is not widely used now.

*Surface therapy.* P-32 can be used for surface intra-cavitary radiation of internal serous surfaces (as colloidal chromic phosphate) in exactly the same way as radio-gold – see below.

For external surfaces, as a beta-ray applicator, it has now been replaced by strontium.

## Radioactive gold

Au-198 (Au is the chemical symbol – Latin 'aurum' = gold) emits mostly betas, plus a small fraction of gamma rays, and has a half-life of 2.7 days (i.e. rather similar to radon's 3.8 days). Penetration is low – less than 50 per cent of the betas reach a third of a millimetre, and none travel over 4 mm. The gammas are far more penetrating, and can be detected and counted externally (as with I-131).

For therapy, it is generally prepared in *colloidal form.* A colloid (Greek 'colla' = glue) differs from an ordinary solution; the molecules are so large that they do not pass freely through the body membranes. A colloid injected at a given site therefore does not move around freely, but tends to stay where it is deposited.

*Therapeutic uses.* Au-198 can be used in two ways:

1. *Intra-cavitary* (beta therapy of internal surfaces) – injection of colloid into cavities (chiefly peritoneal and pleural) to irradiate the serous surfaces in order to inhibit malignant effusion of fluid. It can also be injected into the *bladder* to treat very superficial papillomas.

2. *Interstitial* (gamma therapy as gold grains) – insertion of short lengths of metallic gold, sheathed to absorb the betas.

## Intra-cavitary treatment of peritoneal and pleural effusions

Exudation of fluid from serous surfaces by malignant growth is common in, e.g. lung, breast and ovarian cancer, and causes dyspnoea, abdominal enlargement and discomfort etc. Paracentesis gives relief, but re-accumulation may be rapid, and frequent tappings are inconvenient and exhausting for the patient, especially as considerable loss of protein occurs. External radiation rarely helps, but a radioactive colloid can be injected into the cavity so that the particles are deposited on the serous surfaces and irradiate them.

The deeper tissues of lung or bowel etc. will receive virtually no beta radiation, but only the small fraction of gamma rays, which give a dose insufficient to cause noticeable effects. This method is therefore essentially a form of internal superficial 'bath' therapy. Superficial malignant cells will be destroyed or damaged, surface blood and lymphatic capillaries will be obliterated by the radiation reaction, and a protective layer of scar tissue may form on the surfaces. All these processes will discourage the further formation of fluid. But if there are large masses of growth, this method will fail, as the betas cannot penetrate to influence anything more than about 2 mm deep to the surface.

The procedure is best carried out in the theatre, with full aseptic precautions. The bulk of the fluid exudate is first removed from the pleural or peritoneal cavity, and the gold solution is instilled by gravity feed via the same needle, usually from a special apparatus on which the gold container is mounted in a lead pot, and another container delivers saline to flush the tubing. For a case of ascites, 100-200 mCi are injected; in a pleural cavity, 75-100 mCi.

In abdominal cases with little or no fluid present, a small incision may be made down to the peritoneum, to make sure that the isotope enters the peritoneal cavity (and not the bowel or abdominal wall where it would cause local necrosis).

After the instillation, to ensure uniform bathing of the surfaces, the patient is turned on his back, then on his face, then on each side, then with the pelvis raised. These changes of position are repeated on the ward every half-hour for the next half day.

The nurse should inspect the wound at intervals to see if there is any leakage. Rubber gloves should be worn when dressings are handled. The patient is a source of gamma radiation and nursing procedures should be as expeditious as possible.

Since the colloidal gold particles remain fixed to the pleural or peritoneal surfaces, with very little absorption, there is hardly any radioactive excretion via urine or faeces, and no special precautions are necessary for their disposal. Should death occur soon after instillation, precautions must be taken as detailed on p. 106.

This method is successful in slowing down re-accumulation of fluid in about 50 per cent of cases. Similar success can now be achieved by intra-cavitary instillation of *cytotoxic drugs* (see Chapter 13) and since these involve no radiation hazards, they are now generally preferred. If cytotoxics fail, a radioactive colloid may still succeed.

*Intra-cavitary treatment of papillomatosis of bladder.* Colloidal gold can be introduced into the bladder, via a catheter, for surface irradiation of very superficial multiple papillomata, and it is possible to clear the bladder lining in this way.

Similar results are also obtainable by intra-vesical cytotoxic drugs – e.g. thiotepa (p. 224).

*Gold grains.* Short lengths (2 mm) of gold wire are inserted into fine platinum tubes. These 'grains' are activated in the nuclear reactor to a strength of about 1 or 2 mCi. The platinum filters off the betas, so the effective radiation is gamma alone. They are inserted by a special introducer, a gold-grain 'gun' (Fig. 11.4) which has a magazine into which the grains are loaded. The whole instrument can be sterilized by dry heat in an autoclave.

Gold grains are used e.g. in bladder implants (p. 156) and in Britain *have now entirely replaced radon seeds.*

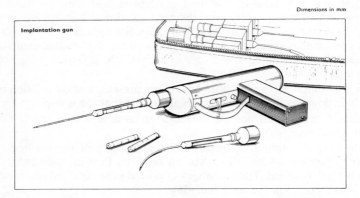

Fig. 11.4 Implantation gun and magazines for gold grains. (Medical Supply Association Ltd.)

## Radioactive yttrium

Y-90 emits betas only, and has a half-life of 2.5 days. They are more energetic than the betas of gold; 50% travel 1 mm, and the maximum range is 10 mm.

*Uses*

(1) *Intra-cavitary.* Compounds of yttrium, including colloidal solutions, have been used in the same way as radio-gold, for control of malignant effusions.

(2) *Interstitial,* especially for destruction of the pituitary gland, in hormonal treatment of (mostly) breast cancer (see p. 213). It is inserted either as tiny pellets or as a rod; or as a paste packed into the pituitary fossa after surgical hypophysectomy, to destroy remnants of the gland which can never be completely removed by the surgeon.

## Radioactive strontium

Sr-90 has a half-life of 28 years, and emits betas only. Depth-dosage is shown in Fig. 11.5 — it falls off very rapidly.

*Use.* Its chief use is as a *beta-ray source for surface application, especially on the eye.* The applicator is like a contact lens, curved to fit the surface of the eyeball. Strontium foil is mounted just beneath the concave surface, and backed by silver foil which absorbs the betas emitted in the backward direction.

The eye is anaesthetised, and the applicator is either slipped under the eyelids or held in position by hand or forceps for the few minutes needed for each treatment.

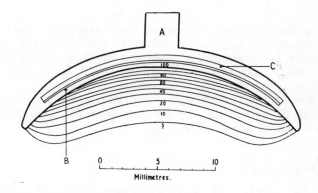

Fig. 11.5 Diagram of strontium foil applicator, with depth isodose contours. A, plastic, B, active foil, C, silver foil. (*Sinclair and Trott, British Journal of Radiology*)

*Corneal vascularisation.* The normal cornea is completely devoid of blood vessels. Ulcers or infections may lead to abnormal extension of tiny vessels from the marginal conjunctiva to heal the lesion (Fig. 11.6), but the new vessels are liable to persist, even after their purpose has been served, and with them any corneal scar is liable to persist also. If they can be obliterated, fading of the corneal opacity is encouraged. Localised radiation can produce a reaction that seals the vessels, and this is the object of therapy. Small leashes of vessels can be treated by weekly applications.

*Corneal grafts.* An opaque cornea can be excised surgically and replaced by another cornea. The success of the graft is liable to be marred by ingrowing blood vessels from the margin, leading to opacifica-

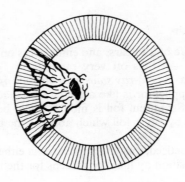

Fig. 11.6 Vascularisation in corneal ulcer.

tion of the grafted cornea. To irradiate these vessels, an annular source (Latin 'annulus' = ring) of strontium is used. Treatment may be pre-operative, post-operative, or both, and can make all the difference between failure and success. A typical course is of four weekly applications, giving 600 rads at the surface each time.

*Neoplasms.* It is occasionally possible to treat a small neoplasm on the conjunctiva, e.g. melanoma – by a strontium plaque, 2500 rads once a week to a total of about 15000 rads.

## Radioactive iridium

Ir-192 has a half-life of 74 days, and emits betas and gammas.

It has been used in a gamma ray beam unit, like cobalt, but the short half-life necessitates frequent recharging in the nuclear reactor, which must therefore be within reasonable distance.

It has also been used as a radium substitute, e.g. in a vaginal applicator in treatment of the cervix. The softer gamma rays make it easier to protect the rectum and bladder as compared with radium, and simplifies protection problems generally – just as with caesium (see p. 56).

Iridium wire can also be used, sheathed in platinum tubing (like gold grains) which absorbs the betas. This gives us a gamma-ray source that can substitute for radium.

The wire is flexible and can easily be bent into any required shape, and cut into convenient lengths. Its use in interstitial treatment of bladder cancer is described on p. 156. It has also been used for awkward sites such as the back of the tongue and the anal canal, where its easy adaptability in length and curvature is advantageous. Small ring-shaped applicators have also been useful on the eyeball etc.

It is also useful in *after-loading* techniques (compare p. 56). Plastic

tubes are first inserted, e.g. for a growth in the mouth, and these are
checked radiographically. If the layout is satisfactory, iridium wire is
then threaded into the tubes.

# 12. Hormones in Cancer Therapy

*Yet nature is made better by no mean*
*But nature makes that mean.*

Shakespeare (The Winter's Tale)

## Historical development

The relationship between hormones and tumours is not a new concept. An early milestone was the work of a Scottish surgeon Beatson in 1896 (i.e. about the same time as the discovery of X-rays and radium). Basing himself on veterinary work on cows which demonstrated a relation between the ovary and milk production, he removed the ovaries of two young women with breast tumours and found the tumours then regressed. It was thought at the time that the mechanism involved removal of some 'ovarian irritation' responsible for the breast lesions, but recurrence soon took place, and though others repeated the procedure, the results were irregular and improvements only temporary, so that the operation fell into disuse and its full significance was not appreciated.

Later animal work drew attention again to hormonal factors, e.g. the incidence of spontaneous breast cancer in mice was reduced by ovariectomy. Other striking experiments produced breast tumours in mice by prolonged administration of ovarian hormones. Clinical interest revived when in 1941 Huggins in U.S.A. reported the favourable results of orchidectomy on cancer of the prostate, and a spate of work has followed ever since, involving the hormonal activity of the gonads, adrenals, pituitary, thyroid, etc.

Experimental induction of neoplasia by endocrine manipulation can easily be achieved in laboratory animals. The essential mechanism seems to be a *prolonged overstimulation of the target tissue* by virtue of its physiological action, and not by acting as a crude irritant like a carcinogenic chemical. We cannot apply the results of these experiments directly to human cancer, since the experimental endocrine disturbances are more severe and prolonged than ever occurs in humans.

Of human cancers, hormones seem likely to be somehow involved in those of the prostate, breast, uterus, thyroid and possibly kidney. Many other organs are governed by hormones – e.g. ovary, testis, adrenals – but hormone therapy has so far not been found to influence any growths of these tissues.

## Hormones as therapeutic agents

It is a most remarkable fact that hormones should be able to influence an established cancer at all. It seems to run counter to the conventional idea of cancer as a completely independent growth process, 'running wild' and submitting to no restraint. This is of the greatest interest and importance to modern theories of the essential nature of cancer, and we now regard the boundary between cancer and non-cancer as very much less clear-cut than we used to think.

There are only a few human cancers where hormone therapy is of practical value, and these are in organs where hormonal stimulation and control is known to be important – mainly prostate, breast, thyroid and body of uterus – and only a modest proportion of these do actually respond as a rule. Remissions, when they occur, may last for weeks, months or (exceptionally) years, and the relief in patients who do respond may be substantial and even dramatic.

Hormone therapy is superior to surgery, radiation or cytotoxic drugs, in that it does no significant damage to normal tissues and is capable of influencing widely disseminated growths.

Unfortunately, the effects are *temporary, never permanent,* the growth escapes eventually from control, and recurrence sooner or later is inevitable. Moreover, hormone therapy is almost always accompanied by unwanted *side-effects,* which are sometimes objectionable and may even be dangerous. Clearly we have to balance these against the potential benefits, and in practice it may be necessary to stop treatment because of this.

Hormone therapy involves changing the existing hormonal pattern or balance in a patient. There are, broadly, two main ways of achieving this:

1. *Addition* – administration of hormone preparations, by oral or intramuscular (I.M.) route.

2. *Subtraction* – surgical removal or radiation inhibition of endocrine glands, to remove the supply of particular hormones.

## Addition of hormones

*1. Female hormones* of ovarian origin:

a. *Oestrogen* – i.e. oestrus-producing (oestrus is heat or sexual impulse in female mammals). It is responsible for enlargement of breasts at puberty and at menstrual cycles, and for maturation and maintenance of secondary sexual characters and sexual organs.

b. *Progestogen* – its primary function is to maintain the uterus with its implanted fertilised egg during the early months of pregnancy.

*Oestrogens.* Preparations include:

Stilboestrol – the most frequently used of all, a synthetic oestrogen. Five milligrams t.i.d. (Latin *ter in die* = thrice in the day, or t.d.s. – *ter* (in) *die sumendum* = to be taken thrice daily).

Ethinyl oestradiol (0.1 mg t.i.d.) – one of several preparations alternative to stilboestrol.

Premarin – brand name of a preparation of natural oestrogens, derived from pregnant mares' urine (1.25 mg t.i.d.). Useful if others cause sickness.

*Side-effects of oestrogens* occur in a third of patients:

a. Nausea and vomiting – especially from stilboestrol.

b. Fluid retention – which can precipitate pulmonary oedema and congestive heart failure; a low-salt diet helps to combat this.

c. Enlargement of breasts.

d. Deepening of pigmentation of nipple and areola.

e. Uterine bleeding, from stimulation of the endometrium, even long after the menopause. This is also liable to occur if the oestrogen is stopped abruptly; dosage should be tapered off gradually. The patient should always be warned of possible bleeding to avoid alarm.

f. Hypercalcaemia (in excess of the normal 9-11 mg per 100 ml), due to increased mobilisation of calcium from bone. This can also occur apart from oestrogen therapy. It causes decreased neuromuscular excitability, with weakness, anorexia, constipation and generalised pain. The pathology is obscure, there may or may not be osteolytic secondaries, and it is possible that the growth itself produces a substance which acts like parathyroid hormone in releasing calcium from bone. At high levels (16-20 mg), fatal coma and anuria can result.

*Progestogens.* Preparations include:

Hydroxyprogesterone (Primolut-Depot), 250 mg I.M., thrice weekly.

Medroxyprogesterone (Provera), 50 mg I.M. daily, or 100 mg tablets orally four times a day.

Norethisterone (SH420) – 10 mg oral t.i.d.

*Side-effects* – fluid retention is possible.

2. *Male hormones or androgens* (Greek 'andro' = man) which cause masculinisation. Preparations include:

Testosterone propionate – 100 mg I.M., thrice weekly.

Fluoxymesterone (Ultandren) – 10 mg orally t.i.d.

*Side-effects*: fluid retention; virilisation after three months on treatment, especially hirsutism (growth of hair on face etc.), deepening of voice, increased libido.

Androgens also have a protein-anabolic action and the allied anabolic steroids also have some androgenic effects:

Nandrolone phenylpropionate (Durabolin) – 25-50 mg I.M. weekly.

Nandrolone decanoate (Deca-durabolin) – 50 mg I.M. every two or three weeks.

Drostanolone (Masteril) – 100 mg I.M. weekly.

3. *Adrenal hormones* have complicated effects on electrolyte and water balance, carbohydrate and protein metabolism. They are called *corticosteroids* (from adrenal cortex).

In cancer therapy the most commonly used preparations are:

Prednisone and Prednisolone − 20-30 mg daily in divided oral doses. Dexamethasone − 1.5 mg orally t.i.d. (less commonly used).

*Side-effects* are important and potentially serious, especially after prolonged dosage:

a. Exaggeration of normal physiological action, causing hypertension, muscle weakness, diabetes, fluid retention and a Cushing-type syndrome including 'mooning' of the face due to local oedema.

b. Euphoria − a mild degree of this is valuable, but there may be more serious mental disturbance, especially with a past history of mental disorder.

c. Modification of tissue reactions, resulting in spread of infections, or failure of wound or ulcer healing − e.g. haemorrhage or perforation may occur from a peptic ulcer.

d. Osteoporosis, especially in the elderly, which may cause e.g. vertebral collapse.

Note − patients on steroids should carry cards giving details of drugs and dosage and possible complications. Long-term therapy leads to atrophy of the adrenal cortex. This is potentially dangerous, since the adrenals can no longer react to stress by increased hormone secretion, and any acute infection, injury etc. can lead to a state of collapse like an Addisonian crisis. Increased doses must be given in these circumstances, including operative procedures.

*4. Thyroid hormone* − see pp. 196, and 214.

## Subtraction of hormones

### 1. Ovaries

The chief source of female hormone may be removed surgically − *oophorectomy* (ovariectomy), which is usually a minor procedure, necessitating only a few days in hospital. Alternatively, the secretory activity of the ovaries can be suppressed by a sterilisation dose of X-rays (as for menorrhagia − p. 248); this is simpler, but has the drawback that it takes about three months to become effective.

### 2. Testes

The male hormone can be simply abolished by bilateral *orchidectomy*.

### 3. Adrenals

The glands may be removed by surgical *adrenalectomy*. If large enough doses of corticosteroids are given (cortisone, prednisone etc.), the glands will atrophy from disuse and this is tantamount to a *medical adrenalectomy*.

### 4. Pituitary

This is the master endocrine gland, as it controls all the others by its various secretions (Fig. 12.1). Its removal leads to atrophy of ovaries, adrenals, thyroid etc. This may be achieved (though not perfectly) by surgical hypophysectomy, or the gland may be destroyed by radiation. High dosage is required, which can be attained only by interstitial methods, e.g. gold grains, or an yttrium rod.

These can be inserted transnasally, with the help of radiographic control with a fluorescent screen. It is a much less formidable procedure than resection, and can be tolerated by a patient unfit for surgery (Fig. 12.2).

When the gland is destroyed, some of the missing hormones – especially cortisone and thyroxine – must be supplied artificially for the rest of the patient's life.

### Hormone therapy in breast cancer

The normal breast is subject to cyclical growth changes at every monthly cycle and every pregnancy. These are responses to controlled stimulation by hormones of ovary, pituitary and adrenals (Fig. 12.1). Whatever the role of hormones may be in the causation of breast cancer – and we know very little about this – there is no doubt about their effectiveness in treatment in many cases.

Hormone therapy is generally reserved for treatment of the late or recurrent case, especially where dissemination has taken place. In practice, *two-thirds of all cases require palliative treatment for the later stages.*

For local palliation of metastases causing symptoms – especially

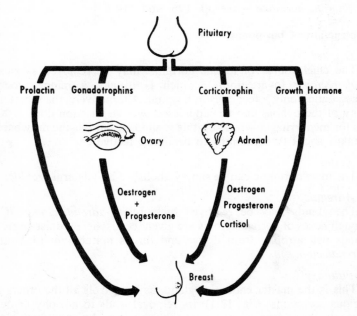

Fig. 12.1 The hormonal control of the normal breast (*Courtesy Prof. Forrest, in Pye's Surgical Handicraft, Wright*)

secondaries in bone – radiation is more effective and should be used. Palliative surgery may also have a place – e.g. for recurrent nodules in the skin flaps, or operable masses of cancer in the breast itself. We *resort to hormones when disease becomes too extensive or generalised*. There are exceptions to this rule – e.g. in an elderly patient we may prefer to begin with hormone treatment, even for a localised growth, since many growths at this age respond well, and it may be less of a strain than surgery or radiation.

## Choice of hormonal method

In general, we begin with the simpler methods first and, if the treatment causes improvement, use it until the growth escapes from control – as it always does eventually. Then we turn to another method in the light of the previous response (or lack of response) and such factors as age, general condition, etc. When the time comes to consider the more drastic methods of operative ablation, we must carefully weigh the reasonable expectation of life against the inevitable discomforts of treatment – and the price will often be judged too high.

Unfortunately there is no simple test available to indicate the probable response of a particular patient to treatment, or to pick out the best hormone to use. It is therefore usually a matter of trial and error. Various biochemical tests have been investigated, but none is of great value. One test which has its advocates is the *Discriminant Function*. This is based on estimations of hormones in the patient's urine, and a mathematical formula is applied to give a numerical result; a strong positive points to probable hormone dependence.

## First-line treatment

In the first instance, the best guide is the patient's ovarian hormone status:
1. Pre-menopausal.
2. Late post-menopausal, i.e. 10 years or more after the menopause.
3. Early post-menopausal.

1. In pre-menopausal patients, *therapeutic castration* is the first line in hormonal management. Surgical *oophorectomy* is best, especially if there is any urgency (e.g. multiple bone secondaries, involvement of brain or liver) or if growth is rapid. *Radiation castration* (as described on p. 248) is an effective alternative but takes 2-3 months to work, and this delay is usually undesirable.

This method succeeds in relieving 20-30 per cent of cases and the remission may last for up to two years. Bone pain is usually relieved, often quite dramatically, and osteolytic lesions may recalcify. Soft tissue lesions usually respond less well.

*Medical castration* by administration of androgenic hormones is a possible alternative but gives inferior results.

2. In late post-menopausal patients, *oestrogens* are first choice – usually stilboestrol if tolerated. In the older patients (60+) the response is

often very gratifying, and a large breast mass may melt away and ulceration heal. Bone secondaries respond less well. Good response occurs in a third of cases; the longer the time since the menopause, the more likely is oestrogen to succeed.

Remission may last up to 18 months.

3. In early post-menopausal patients, the problem is more difficult, since the hormone status is more uncertain. Up to two years after the menopause, *oophorectomy* should still be advised, since some oestrogen continues to be produced by the ovaries. An indication of this can be obtained by cytological examination of a vaginal smear.

Between two and five years after the menopause, *androgen therapy* should be used. After the fifth year, oestrogens should be given first.

*Second-line treatment*

When the effect of the above first-line treatment has worn off, and reactivation of growth occurs – or if the treatment fails completely after a trial of 1-2 months – we can fall back on second lines:

1. Administration of hormones – androgens, corticosteroids, progestogens.

2. Endocrine ablation – adrenalectomy, hypophysectomy, pituitary implantation.

*Androgens.* If there has already been a good response to castration, androgen therapy will yield a useful improvement in 30 per cent of cases. But if castration has failed, it is unlikely to help.

Where there has previously been a good response to oestrogens, androgen therapy can relieve 20 per cent of cases.

*Corticosteroids* are valuable even if sex hormone therapy fails. They can give striking relief of bone pain, and are indicated for hypercalcaemia and secondaries in lung, liver and brain. The increased feeling of well-being is also useful. If the patient is too ill for endocrine surgery, steroids are generally indicated.

*Progestogens* may be useful for soft tissue deposits, but rarely improve bone or visceral deposits. If sex hormone therapy has failed, they are a possible alternative to steroids.

In general, the important thing seems to be to *change the hormonal environment* of the growth and this is probably more important than the precise nature of the hormone used. If a growth responds to, say, oestrogen and eventually begins to grow again, further improvement may sometimes be obtained simply by withdrawing the oestrogen. When further activation of growth occurs later, another useful response may follow administration of oestrogen again.

**Endocrine ablation**

*Adrenalectomy* (bilateral) is particularly useful if there has been a good previous response to castration, and is more effective than medical suppression with steroids.

*Hypophysectomy* is also likely to be useful if castration has been effective. The choice between adrenalectomy and hypophysectomy will depend on local experience and the availability of interested surgeons.

Successful remissions are obtained in 30 per cent of treated cases. But the mortality rate is high, 10-15 per cent.

*Pituitary implantation,* e.g. by radioactive yttrium (Fig. 12.2) is a less severe procedure and may succeed even if there has been no useful response to previous hormone therapy.

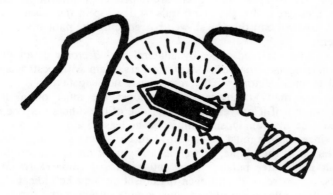

Fig. 12.2 An yttrium rod implanted in the pituitary through a screw-type trocar. (*Courtesy Prof. Forrest in Pye's Surgical Handicraft, Wright*)

Major endocrine surgery has had a considerable vogue in various places, but enthusiasm is declining. Useful results are certainly obtainable in a modest proportion of cases, but the price is high and the quality of remaining life is always doubtful.

### Cancer of the male breast

The best form of hormone therapy is surgical castration, the relatively simple procedure of bilateral *orchidectomy*. This is effective in two-thirds of cases, a remarkably high proportion, and double the success rate of oestrogen therapy or oophorectomy in females.

Oestrogen therapy succeeds in only about 15 per cent and is therefore not the method of first choice.

Radiation castration is not practicable in the male. When tumour control ceases after orchidectomy, steroid therapy is more likely to help than adrenalectomy or hypophysectomy.

*Summary conclusion*

Hormone therapy is a palliative for advanced and disseminated breast cancer, and is effective only in a minority of cases (20-30 per cent). The average period of control in successful cases is 1-2 years and the quality of life can be good. More than one method can be used in sequence.

The more drastic methods of endocrine ablation should be applied only to very carefully selected cases, after weighing up all the factors.

**Cancer of the prostate** (see also p. 166).

This is one of the commonest cancers in men (Table 1.2, p. 8). Radical prostatectomy is seldom possible, as few patients are seen early enough. Hormone therapy is therefore the treatment of most cases, and fortunately 90 per cent of prostatic cancers are dependent on hormone stimulation, i.e. androgens, for the gland fails to develop in the absence of androgens. Growth can thus be slowed by reducing the patient's supply of androgens.

This can be achieved either by bilateral *orchidectomy* or administration of *oestrogens* − or both. Most workers begin with oestrogens and proceed to orchidectomy if the response is not satisfactory.

There are many oestrogen preparations; the most often used is Stilboestrol, but if it proves nauseating, one of the others may be better tolerated (see above). Dosage must be at least 5 mg t.d.s. and often higher, since enough must be given to cause mammary enlargement and pigmentation of the nipple, as well as atrophy of the testis. Interference with salt and water balance may cause cardiac embarrassment, and diuretics, a salt-free diet and even digitalisation may be indicated. Hormone treatment usually results in considerable softening and shrinkage of the growth, with relief of symptoms.

When primary hormone therapy fails, relief can often be obtained by corticosteroids, and this is in practice likely to be more effective than adrenalectomy. Apart from hormone therapy, good palliative relief of obstructive symptoms is available from transurethral resection. Painful secondary deposits are common, especially in pelvic and vertebral bones. These may respond to localised external radiation, but not as reliably as breast cancer secondaries.

Since megavoltage is now more widely available, there is a revival of interest in high-dose irradiation of the primary growth, and good palliation of bladder-neck obstruction can be obtained by small-field beam--directed external radiation.

**Cancer of the thyroid**

Hormone therapy has been discussed on p. 196.

The standard dosage of thyroxine is 0.1 mg t.d.s. but must be controlled by observation of pulse rate etc. An alternative drug is liothyronine (T3 − 20 $\mu$g 8 hourly). Its onset and decline of action is more rapid, and this makes it more suitable if thyroid scanning is to be undertaken, since a scan can be made a week after the drug is stopped, whereas a delay of three weeks is necessary when thyroxine is used.

## Cancer of body of uterus

The endometrium is another tissue subject to hormonal control, and some cases of uncontrolled cancer of the uterine body may benefit from *progestogen* therapy (see above, p. 208).

## Cancer of the kidney

The kidney and uterus are related embryologically, both being derived from the 'urogenital ridge'. This helps to explain why, in some cases, *progestogens* can help in advanced renal cancer.

# 13. Cytotoxic Chemotherapy

*Not for the good that it will do,*
*But that nothing may be left undone*
*On the margin of the impossible.*

T.S. Eliot (The Family Reunion)

This form of treatment is termed *cytotoxic* (Greek for 'cell poisoning') or *oncolytic* (Greek 'oncos' = tumour, 'lytic' = dissolving or destroying).

The modern story goes back no further than the 1930s, with the chemical identification of carcinogenic substances present in tar. Soon after came the discovery that these substances could also *inhibit* the growth of normal and cancer tissues – just as X-rays and radium can be both destructive of all growth and carcinogenic. This chemical clue was followed up by testing allied chemical compounds on animal tumours in the laboratory. The turning point came during the Second World War, from the investigation of poison gases. (Even during the First World War; sulphur 'mustard' gas, was seen to have, apart from its vesicant action on the skin, severe depressant effect on bone marrow, and leucopenia was noted in those dying of mustard gas). War gases were studied again, and in the 1940's the nitrogen 'mustards' were found to cause gene mutations and chromosome damage leading to cell death at subsequent mitosis – just like radiation. These agents are therefore *radio-mimetic* (i.e. radiation-imitating). Profound effects were observed on the marrow, and cautious trials were begun on cancers involving marrow, with some encouraging results. The stage was now clearly set, and research has since proceeded with gathering momentum. Many thousands of complex chemical compounds have been synthesised and tested on animals. Only a few have proved of value in human cancer, but a new chapter has been opened.

*Medical oncology* is virtually a new department, and cytotoxic chemotherapy now takes its place alongside surgery and radiotherapy as one of the three major agents in cancer therapy. Some doctors now specialise in medical oncology, just as others do in surgical or radiation oncology. In many centres, chemotherapy is practised also by radiotherapists, haematologists, surgeons, physicians and others, depending on local interests and resources.

The subject is new, and current developments rapid. Inevitably and properly, progress had to be cautious and tentative, after experimental work on animals. Trials could be justified only on patients who had failed to respond to established methods (surgery and/or radiation). With increased experience, it became justifiable to use these drugs at earlier stages.

## General principles and side-effects

As the epithet 'cell poisonous' implies, these drugs interfere drastically and, as a rule, indiscriminately with all growth and mitosis – much like radiation. They are *not specific* to cancers in general or any cancer in particular, and cannot be compared with, e.g. antibiotics which are lethal to particular organisms without damaging the tissues.

It follows that *they are no substitute for surgery or radiotherapy* where these are known to be effective, and are, in general, used where *surgery and radiation have either failed or are not applicable.* Their range of application is not as wide as that of radiation, and many (in fact, most) growths are unresponsive to the maximum tolerable doses of cytotoxic drugs.

In only a few instances are they the *treatment of choice* from the start, e.g.:

| | |
|---|---|
| Choriocarcinoma ⎫<br>Burkitt's lymphoma ⎭ | In these two, cytotoxics can be genuinely curative. |
| Leukaemia | Most forms. |
| Myelomatosis | Many cases. |
| Teratoma of testis ⎫<br>Wilms's embryoma<br>of kidney ⎬<br>Neuroblastoma ⎭ | In combination with surgery and/or radiation. |

In some departments it is, or was, true that cytotoxic therapy tends to be reserved only – or mainly – for the late and hopeless case, sometimes as a gesture to solace the patient or relative, that 'everything possible is being done'. This may have been reasonable years ago when the subject was in its infancy, but we now have enough knowledge to make the therapy more rational and scientific.

Any drug can be misused, and until experience is gained it is virtually inevitable that it will be wrongly used at the start. Dosage and timing are of critical importance, just as in radiotherapy. The 'harmless' aspirin tablets that the public consumes by the ton, can be lethal when a child finds a bottle and helps himself too liberally. Most modern drugs are potent and dangerous and also have unpleasant side-effects; they must be strictly controlled if they are to do more good than harm. Cytotoxic drugs are also potent and dangerous, and we are only slowly learning how to use them to achieve the maximum useful effect with the minimum harm and discomfort. But we *are* learning, and our patients are reaping the benefit. Until recent years, cytotoxics were really useful only in leukaemia and some lymphomas, i.e. growths of scattered or disseminated type. It still remains true that *most of the 'solid' common tumours* (e.g. lung, colon, stomach, cervix) *are not usually responsive to current chemotherapy.* But we are now seeing increasing success in prolonging life and comfort and improving the prognosis generally, in many cancers, where formerly little could be offered.

*Mode of action.* The ideal drug would be one which killed only cancer cells and spared normal tissues completely. This is no more possible (at least yet) than it is with radiation. The most important effect of the drugs in use is on cell mitosis, by interference with the synthesis or functioning of vital nuclear constituents – DNA, RNA, nucleic acids, proteins. They are therefore toxic to all cells, malignant or normal – just like radiation. Their use in cancer depends on the fact that conditions of growth in a cancer are abnormal. The cells of a particular cancer *may* have some inherent chemosensitivity, or they *may* go into mitosis more frequently than their normal counterparts. However, many (even most) cancers do not proliferate faster than normal tissues – many in fact grow more slowly. *But they are less capable than normal tissues of repairing cell damage, so that normal cells can recover while cancer cells do not; this is probably the most important factor of all.* Their effects will thus be comparable to Fig. 5.5 p. 80.

As with radiation, a given dose kills a certain fixed proportion of cells of a tumour mass irrespective of the actual number of cells present. Just as much of the drug will therefore be needed to kill a few cells in a small tumour as to kill many cells in a large mass. Treatment must therefore be continued long after a growth is no longer detectable clinically. At the present time it is not possible to eradicate most 'solid' cancers by drugs, for several reasons – (a) inherent resistance of the cells, (b) failure of the drugs to reach all the cancer cells, (c) our ignorance of just how long treatment should be continued, (d) toxic side effects which set a limit to dosage.

*Dosage and toxicity.* Since the effects are indiscriminate, all tissues are bound to be more or less affected. But damage to normal tissues can be minimised, just as we have learned to do in radiotherapy. Intermittent administration of high doses of drugs will result in stepwise permanent losses of tumour cells, while normal tissues still retain their powers of recovery. This is better than continuous therapy with small doses of drugs, which used to be practised. Low doses are harmful as they accelerate drug resistance (which in any case always occurs eventually) by eliminating the more sensitive cells and leaving the most resistant cells to flourish. It is therefore of vital importance to appreciate the possible toxic effects and balance them against the potential benefit.

The cellular damage, at therapeutic levels, shows itself only when the cell goes into mitosis – or attempts to – just as in the case of radiation. *Rapidly growing normal tissues are therefore affected at least as much as – and usually more than – the cancer itself, and it is this fact that sets the limit to practical therapy.* These tissues include:

1. Haemopoietic tissue, especially bone marrow.

2. Mucous membranes, especially bowel.

3. Hair and skin.

These are the chief limiting factors in actual therapy.

4. Gonads – ovary and testis.
5. The reticulo-endothelial cells responsible for the immune response.

When high-dose treatment is given, patients should be in hospital, and examined daily for toxic effects. Frequent blood counts – haemoglobin, total red and white cells, differential count if indicated, and platelets – should be charted. High fluid intake should be maintained, to avoid bladder damage from products of the drug excreted in the urine, and to remove the excess uric acid produced by rapid cell breakdown in the tumour. Hyperuricaemia can be countered by allopurinol.

*Bone marrow.* Most cytotoxic drugs have profound and critical effects on the rapidly dividing normal marrow tissue, and the resultant deficiencies in red and white cells and platelets can readily lead to anaemia, haemorrhage, infection and death. Polymorph levels of 1000 or less can be tolerated for a week or so. Platelet counts should not be allowed to fall from the norm of 200 000 to much below 80 000.

Severe anaemia and thrombocytopenia (i.e. platelet deficiency) should be corrected by blood transfusion. Antibiotics may be indicated for infection, actual or threatened, but there is always some risk of 'opportunistic' secondary fungal infection, which can be devastating.

Sterile isolation units are not necessary for most regimes but may be justifiable for special cases e.g. choriocarcinoma or leukaemia.

### Mucous membranes

The gastro-intestinal – including oral – mucosa is commonly affected, and the chief clinical result is *diarrhoea* – especially with drugs like 5-fluorouracil, which are known to have early effects on bowel.

With antimetabolite drugs, especially methotrexate, *ulceration in the mouth* is often the first sign of toxicity and may occur the next day. The ulcers are typically on the lip margins, shallow and often painful.

*Bladder ulceration* with haematuria may occur, especially with cyclophosphamide.

### Skin and hair

*Alopecia* is particularly associated with cyclophosphamide; it also occurs with adriamycin, methotrexate etc. Hair grows again after the end of treatment, or even if treatment continues at lower dosage. For women patients, it is a good idea to supply a wig early in the course.

Skin rashes occasionally appear. Erythema may develop in an involved area, e.g. in local infusions or perfusions.

### Gonads

Spermatogenesis is repressed in men. In women, prolonged treatment can cause amenorrhoea. Cytotoxic drugs should not be used in pregnancy, especially in the first four months when there is a high risk of abortion and foetal abnormalities. Gene mutations, inherited by offspring, are a potential hazard.

*Nervous system*

Nausea and vomiting are common, especially after intravenous injections. Anti-emetic drugs, e.g. perphenazine (Fentazin), prochlorperazine (Stemetil) etc. – given an hour beforehand, are helpful.

Neurotoxicity is especially marked with vincristine – see p. 226.

*Immunosuppresion.* Cytotoxics are used for deliberate suppression of the immune response on special occasions, e.g. surgical transplants of kidneys, etc. They can diminish patients' ability to react to infections. The significance of this in cancer is obscure. Some workers are worried that they may damage the body's defence mechanisms against cancer, but the whole subject of the immunology of cancer is so complicated and doubtful that it is impossible to be dogmatic. All treatments carry potential dangers, and risks have always to be carefully balanced.

*Other toxic effects* include:

Adriamycin and Daunorubicin are toxic to the heart beyond a certain level of total dosage (about 600 mg).

Bleomycin can cause dangerous lung fibrosis, and skin changes. Busulphan can cause lung fibrosis and skin pigmentation. Steroids lead to salt and water retention, and can cause diabetes.

*Resistance* to cytotoxics develops eventually – just as it does to antibiotics – and when any member of a group of drugs ceases to be effective, resistance extends to all the other members of the same group. But there may still be a good response to another group. To minimise the effects of resistance, modern *combination therapy* has been developed, using two or more drugs together or in sequence. Recent revolutionary advances have depended largely on this kind of combined attack, and the use of single agents is now not usually justifiable.

Anaplastic growths would be expected to be more susceptible to cytotoxic attack than well-differentiated growths, but this is not necessarily so in practice, possibly owing to the differential development of resistant cells after therapy.

Large tumour masses respond poorly, because of impaired blood supply at the centre – comparable again to radiation.

The best indication and justification for cytotoxic therapy is the presence of *widespread malignancy. Since so many cases, though clinically localised, are actually widely disseminated at the time of diagnosis, it is not surprising that these drugs are assuming ever increasing importance in oncological management.* The correct combination of surgery, radiotherapy and chemotherapy is of literally vital importance. We have still a lot to learn, but progress is definite and encouraging.

## Classification of cytotoxic drugs

The available agents may be divided into the following groups:
1. Alkylating agents

2. Antimetabolites.
3. Plant products. ⎫
                          chromosome inhibitors
4. Antibiotics.      ⎭
5. Miscellaneous.

Details of dosage, routes of administration, etc. are given in Table 13.1.

Doses are approximate, and must always be guided by the blood count and clinical condition.

## 1. Alkylating agents

Alkyl is the name of the chemical group common to the alcohols – hence the name *Alkylation* refers to the chemical process of combination of the alkyl group with various chemical groups of biological importance in cells. These include protein constituents and precursors, especially of the cell nucleus, and the result is gross interference with their functioning in mitosis etc.

These agents are all chemically related to mustard gas – hence the name of the first useful substance developed, *Mustine*. The most commonly used members of the group are listed in Table 13.1

*Mustine* is still one of the most effective of all cytotoxic drugs. It is unstable, and should be dissolved immediately before injection. Like mustard gas, it is intensely vesicant and irritant to tissues. If injected outside a vein, local pain and possibly necrosis result. Phlebitis and thrombosis may be caused, and the drug is therefore often injected into the tubing of a saline infusion, though this is not essential for the experienced doctor. Nausea and vomiting nearly always follow within a few hours. To counter this, 50 mg chlorpromazine (Largactil) and 90 mg phenobarbitone may be given an hour beforehand and at four-hourly intervals for the next 24 hr. The injection is best given in the evening, followed by a sedative for the night. Most patients, however, receive injections as out--patients during the day.

Late effects include epilation and temporary amenorrhoea. Excessive dosage leads to anaemia, thrombocytopenia, fever and bleeding, which can be fatal. The white cell count begins to fall almost from the start, is at its lowest after a week, and takes about six weeks to recover.

*Chief uses:*

a. Reticuloses – especially Hodgkin's in later stages (see p. 179). Rapid relief may be obtained in acute toxic cases and severe systemic symptoms may be controlled much earlier than by radiation. Fever and weakness may subside in a few days, but pruritus is less often relieved.

b. Lung cancer – especially anaplastic (oat-cell) types.

c. Malignant effusions – often effective on intrapleural or intraperitoneal instillation of 20-30 mg (compare radioactive gold, pp. 200-202).

Table 13.1 Cytotoxic agents used in cancer therapy

| Drug | Proprietary name | Administration route and average dosage | Main uses |
|---|---|---|---|
| **Mustine** (Nitrogen mustard) | | I.V. 0.4 mg/kg single dose; or divided, e.g. in four daily fractions. Intra-cavitary, 10-20 mg. | Reticuloses, especially Hodgkin's. Malignant effusions. Other cancers, e.g. lung. |
| **Chlorambucil** | Leukeran | Oral. 0.2 mg/kg daily. Typical initial dose = 10-12 mg. Maintenance, 2-5 mg daily. | Chronic lymphatic leukaemia. Other reticuloses, especially lymphosarcoma, Hodgkin's. Other cancers, e.g. ovary. |
| **Cyclophosphamide** | Endoxan (a) Cytoxan | I.V. 200 mg daily for 10 days. For rapid effect, 500-1000 mg daily to total 3-5 g. Oral (especially maintenance), 50-200 mg daily. | Reticuloses – most types, including Burkitt's. Myelomatosis. Other cancers, e.g. lung, ovary, breast. |
| **Thiophosphoramide** | Thiotepa | I.V. or I.M. 15-30 mg alternate days, to total 150-180 mg; then weekly or fortnightly maintenance. Intra-cavitary, 45-60 mg. | Ovary; breast; malignant effusions. |
| **Melphalan** | Alkeran | Oral. 10 mg daily for 7-10 days. I.V. 50-100 mg weekly. | Myelomatosis; malignant melanoma (limb perfusion). Other cancers, e.g. ovary. |
| **Busulphan** | Myleran | Oral. 2 mg twice or thrice daily. | Chronic myeloid leukaemia. |
| **6-Mercaptopurine** | Puri-nethol | Oral. 2.5 mg/kg daily; adults, 150 mg daily. | Acute leukaemia; Choriocarcinoma. |
| **Methotrexate** | | Oral. 2.5-10 mg, alternate days, until mouth sore. I.V. 2.5-5 mg daily for 2-5 days. Intra-arterial infusion, 50 mg daily for 6-10 days, plus citrovorum factor (I.M. 6 mg four-hourly). | Acute childhood leukaemia. Choriocarcinoma. Burkitt's lymphoma. Infusions – cancers of head and neck, pelvis etc. |

*table contd.*

| Drug | Regime | Indications |
|---|---|---|
| **5-Fluorouracil (5 FU)** | I.V. 15 mg/kg daily for five days, then half dose alternate days until toxicity. | Cancers of gastro-intestinal tract. |
| **Vinblastine** Velbe Velban | I.V. Initially 0.1 mg/kg weekly. Typically, 5-15 mg weekly or fortnightly. | Hodgkin's. Choriocarcinoma. |
| **Vincristine** Oncovin | I.V. 0.01 mg /kg weekly, increasing by 0.01 mg until toxicity. | Acute childhood leukaemia. Some other reticuloses and cancers. |
| **Actinomycin-D** | I.V. 0.01 mg/kg daily for five days. Adults – 1.0 mg daily for 4-5 days. | Wilms's tumour; Teratoma testis; Choriocarcinoma. |
| **Adriamycin** | I.V. children – up to 800 $\mu$g/kg/day. Adults – up to 650 $\mu$g/kg/day. | Acute leukaemia. Childhood tumours. Breast, ovary, teratoma. |
| **Daunorubicin** | I.V. 30-60 mg/m$^2$/day. | Leukaemia. Childhood tumours. |
| **Bleomycin** | I.M. 15 mg daily I.V. 15-30 mg daily | Squamous carcinoma. |
| **L-Asparaginase** | I.V. 200-500 units/kg/day | Acute leukaemia. |
| **Cytosine Arabinoside** Cytarabine | I.V. 2 mg/kg | Acute leukaemia. |
| **Procarbazine** Natulan | Oral. Initially 50 mg, increase by 50 mg daily in divided doses after meals, to maximum daily 4 mg/kg (i.e. 150-300 mg daily) for 21 days. Maintenance, 50 mg daily or alternate days. | Hodgkin's. |

NOTE: All the above regimes are approximate only and always controlled by full blood counts, clinical state and toxicity.

It is particularly useful where speed of action is important – e.g. in mediastinal obstruction or spinal cord compression – especially if radiation is not available; or the two agencies may be combined.

*Chlorambucil* has the advantage of oral administration, though its action is slower than that of mustine. Its effects are similar, but more pronounced on lymphocytes.

*Chief uses:*

a. Reticuloses – especially chronic lympathic leukaemia and lymphosarcoma, which have many similarities and merge into each other.

b. Cancer of ovary, for which it msy be just as good as thiotepa or cyclophosphamide.

*Cyclophosphamide* also has the great advantage of effectiveness by mouth. It is particularly liable to cause *epilation* of the scalp, and somewhat liable to produce sterile cystitis and *bladder ulceration*. These bladder complications can be avoided or minimised by ensuring a high fluid intake. It is the least toxic of the group, and is relatively kind to platelets. Maintenance dosage can be given for many months.

*Chief uses:*

a. Reticuloses – especially myelomatosis, where it is probably as good as melphalan; also useful in Hodgkin's, chronic lymphatic leukaemia, reticulosarcoma.

b. Carcinoma – ovary, breast, lung, etc.

c. Burkitt's tumour – see pp. 233-4.

*Thiotepa* is usually given by intramuscular injection; also into serous cavities for effusions. It may be used for many carcinomas but has been largely superseded.

*Chief uses:*

Cancer of breast and ovary.

*Melphalan* is commonly used for *multiple myeloma*. It has also proved useful in perfusion of upper and lower limbs for malignant melanoma (see below).

*Busulphan* is the best example of preferential action on a particular tissue, since it damages the parent blood cells in *chronic myeloid leukaemia* at lower doses than other cells, so that it is now the treatment of choice and preferable to radiation (see pp. 183-4).

Blood counts should be at least weekly, and dosage continued until the white count is about 20 000 and then stopped – or earlier if platelets fall below 100 000. The count will continue to fall for a time, and the aim should be to stabilise it at around 10 000. Maintenance dosage may then be started and adjusted as the blood count dictates – including the all-important haemoglobin.

Whether this treatment actually prolongs life is uncertain, but it does usually keep the patient symptom-free until near the end and enable him to lead a worthwhile existence.

## 2. Antimetabolites

These are chemical variations of important constituents of cellular metabolism. They act by competing with them in building up nuclear proteins etc. The normal components are 'elbowed out' and the cell forms an abnormal product which is useless for mitosis and so leads to cell death.

*Methotrexate* is usually given orally or intravenously. The typical sign of toxicity is soreness or ulceration in the mouth; alopecia is common. The side-effects can be minimised if the drug is given as an infusion over a period not exceeding 24-36 hours. Toxic effects are more liable after prolonged oral administration.

Its unwanted effects on the body generally can be countered by an antidote – *folinic acid* (also called 'citrovorum factor' or 'leucovorin'), 6 mg intramuscularly, four-hourly. Folinic acid 'rescue' reverses the toxic effect on cells – not on cells which have already been damaged, but it counters the further action of the remainder of the drug which has not yet been excreted. High-dose *pulses* of methotoxate with subsequent rescue are now being used.

Chief uses:
  a. Lymphomas, especially acute leukaemia in children – p. 236.
  b. Choriocarcinoma – p. 232.
  c. Burkitt's tumour – p. 233.
  d. Infusions – cancers of head and neck, and pelvis.

*6-Mercaptopurine (6 MP)* has similarities to methotrexate. It is usually given orally in daily doses. The chief toxic effect is on the marrow, less often on the liver.

Chief uses:
Similar to methotrexate, especially for leukaemias.
It is of little or no value in other malignancies.

*5-Fluorouracil (5 FU)* has been used particularly for *gastrointestinal adenocarcinoma,* and is the only drug that has proved of any value for these.

It is very toxic, with diarrhoea, mouth ulcers, vomiting, alopecia, marrow depression and dermatitis, especially if misused. The first course at least should always be given in hospital. Repeat courses may be given a few weeks later. It is usually given intravenously and is widely used in multi-drug schedules (breast, ovary etc.) It has been given as a hepatic arterial infusion for liver secondaries from the bowel, and some useful results claimed.

Another use is as a local application in ointment form on the skin, to treat superficial hyperkeratoses or basal cell carcinoma recurrent after radiotherapy.

*Cytosine arabinoside (Cytarabine)* is given I.V. and is valuable in acute lymphoblastic leukaemia in children.

*Other antimetabolites* include: thioguanine, hydroxyurea, BCNU, CCNU (nitrosourea compounds).

## 3. Plant products

There are two valuable alkaloids obtained from the periwinkle plant (*vinca rosea*). Their mode of action is unknown.

*Vinblastine* is probably the least toxic agent of all, though great care must be taken to avoid leakage outside the vein, where local necrosis may result.

It is widely used in the later stages of Hodgkins and other lymphomas, and in combination therapy (see below).

*Vincristine* is also widely used in many combinations, for leukaemia (especially acute lymphoblastic), Hodgkin's and other lymphomas, many carcinomas and malignant melanoma and most childhood tumours.

It is a relatively safe drug, though locally irritant. But it is distinguished by its *toxic effect on nerve tissue,* which can be very serious. It causes pain, muscle weakness and atrophy, beginning with foot-drop; also, severe constipation from its effect on the bowel musculature. These effects must be watched for, and the drug must be stopped at the first sign of weakness, or the nerves may not recover. Bulk laxatives (e.g. methyl cellulose) and wetting agents (Dioctyl) should be given.

## 4. Antibiotics

All anti-bacterial agents obtained from fungi etc. are routinely screened for anti-tumour activity in animals. This has led to several valuable products. They act by binding to DNA and so inhibiting it.

*Actinomycin-D* is locally destructive if leaked outside a vein. It can cause nausea and vomiting, marrow depression, sore mouth, alopecia.

*Chief uses:*

a. Childhood tumours – Wilms's tumour, Ewing's tumour, soft tissue sarcomas.

b. Teratoma of testis.

c. Choriocarcinoma.

*Adriamycin* is given intravenously. Toxic effects are – marrow depression, nausea and vomiting, sore mouth, alopecia. A special danger is to the heart – *cardiotoxicity* – so that the total dosage must be strictly limited to 550 mg per square metre of body surface.

It is proving useful in leukaemias, childhood tumours (especially neuroblastoma) and in combinations for many cancers (breast, ovary, etc.)

*Daunorubicin (Daunomycin, Rubidomycin)* is given intravenously. Its toxic effects are very similar to those of adriamycin, including cardiotoxicity. It is of use in leukaemias, and some childhood tumours.

*Bleomycin* differs from other antibotics as it is taken up selectively in relatively high concentration by *squamous tissues,* and also by the lungs.

Its main use is for squamous carcinoma of skin and other structures, e.g. head and neck cancers. Another unusual feature is the *absence of marrow toxicity*, so that the blood picture is not disturbed. It can therefore be used in Hodgkin's disease, etc. when other drugs have failed. It may be given by intramuscular or intravenous route.

Toxic effects are seen on the skin and mouth — swelling, discoloration and hyperkeratosis of hands and fingers, changes over pressure points (knees and elbows), soreness and ulcers in the mouth. A sinister complication is pneumonitis leading to lung fibrosis, which can be fatal. Chest films should be taken at the start and at intervals, and treatment stopped at the first radiological sign of this toxic effect.

## 5. Miscellaneous

There are many other compounds, of which we will describe only a few.

*Corticosteroids* have already been discussed under Hormones (p. 208). In addition to their hormonal effects, they have other actions, including lymphocyte destruction, which are not well understood, but make them of considerable use in some disorders. The best example of this use is in acute leukaemia, especially the lymphoblastic type. They are important constituents of most drug regimes for Hodgkin's and other lymphomas, (e.g. MOPP — see below) and are given orally.

*Procarbazine* is also given by mouth. It can cause nausea and vomiting and some marrow depression and neurological changes. Its action is obscure, and it is of no value in carcinoma. Its chief use is in combination therapy for the lymphomas, (e.g. MOPP).

*L-Asparaginase* is an enzyme, given intravenously. It breaks down asparagine, an amino-acid essential to cell metabolism and growth. Normal cells can synthesise asparagine, but some tumours, especially leukaemias, cannot. The enzyme destroys the amino-acid and so denies it to the cancer cells and causes their death indirectly by deprivation. Its main use is in acute lymphoblastic leukaemia; also in some combination regimes.

*ICRF 159.* This recent *anti-metastatic* drug (initials of Imperial Cancer Research Fund) has only slight cytotoxic action, but acts mainly on the immature blood vessels of a growth, to prevent escape and dissemination of cells, and so reduces the chances of metastasis.

## Localised treatment

When a drug is given by mouth or injection, the whole of the body is exposed to its effects. It would clearly be advantageous to limit its effects to the tumour area if possible, and so spare bone marrow etc. This can be achieved, to some extent at least, in suitable cases by using appropriate routes of administration, in the following ways:

*1. In serous cavities.* Recurrent malignant exudates in the pleural or peritoneal cavity can be treated by exposing the involved walls of the cavity to the drug. The treatment is exactly comparable to the use of radioactive isotopes and since it is a simpler method, involving no radiation hazard, and can give comparable results, it is now generally used as the *first choice in treatment*.

It is injected by needle and syringe into the cavity, after most of the fluid has been removed by aspiration. If the method fails, isotopes can still be tried. Malignant deposits lining the cavity will be attacked directly; some of the drug will be absorbed through the serous membrane and reach the general circulation, but rarely in sufficient quantity to cause serious marrow depression.

The drugs most frequently used are mustine, thiotepa and cyclophosphamide.

*2. In the bladder.* In a comparable way, thiotepa may be injected into the bladder via a catheter, for treatment of multiple papillomatosis. This is again similar to isotope therapy with radio-gold. The solution is left in the bladder for half-an-hour and then withdrawn. The superficial cytotoxic effect can destroy small growths on the bladder lining.

*3. By perfusion.* This is illustrated in Fig. 13.1. If a growth is situated on an extremity (leg, arm or head), the drug can be largely confined to the tumour area by isolating the blood circulation temporarily from the rest of the body. The main artery and vein are exposed surgically and catheterised. The catheters are connected to a motorised pump, and in this way a solution of the drug is pumped through the artery into the tumour area and out again through the vein into the external part of the circuit. This continuous circuit is maintained for about an hour. The

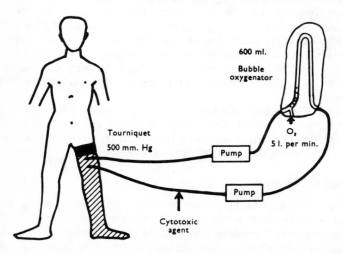

Fig. 13.1 Regional perfusion of a peripheral growth. (*Courtesy Prof. Forrest in Pye's Surgical Handicraft, Wright*)

growth is thus exposed to a high concentration of the drug for a short time, much higher (up to 20 times as high) than can be achieved by oral or intravenous methods, while the rest of the body is largely protected. In practice it is impossible to isolate a part perfectly and there is always a little seepage of the drug into the general circulation, but this is of no serious import.

If the tumour is on a limb, a tourniquet is fastened round the proximal end until the perfusion is over, to achieve more complete isolation from the rest of the body. This technique has proved useful for peripheral *melanoma,* and the best drug here is *melphalan.*

It is a specialised method, and carries appreciable dangers such as bleeding and sepsis post-operatively.

*4. By infusion.* If the tumour area cannot be easily isolated for a perfusion circuit, simple *intra-arterial infusion* can be carried out. A catheter is inserted into the main artery only, either by open exposure or percutaneous puncture. The exact position of the catheter tip and the vascular area served can be ascertained by injecting a radio-opaque contrast medium; adjustments can be made, if necessary, by advancing or retracting the catheter. The extent of skin surface affected can be made visible by injecting a dye (e.g. sulphan blue). The drug is injected through the catheter, either by gravity feed or pump, and almost immediately reaches the tumour region in high concentration. A proportion will, of course, enter the general circulation and produce the usual effects on bone marrow and elsewhere.

The catheter can be maintained in position for many days, and injections made at frequent intervals. Antiseptic precautions are important, as septicaemia is a real threat in a patient whose resistance is likely to be low – as well as thrombosis, peripheral neuritis and haemorrhage.

A recent innovation is to provide a small portable clockwork pump, so that the patient can be ambulant and outside the hospital, and inject the daily dose himself.

The most frequently used drug is *methotrexate,* since its undesirable effects can be countered by the antidote folinic acid.

Unlike perfusion, infusion can be used for e.g. pelvic growths (bladder, cervix, rectum), and even liver and stomach.

*Effect on pain.* Intra-arterial injections often relieve pain, even in the absence of obvious effect on tumour growth. This is due to a direct toxic effect on nerve endings and can be of real clinical value. The action can at times be too pronounced and cause unwanted paraesthesia and even temporary paralysis.

*5. Direct application.* High concentrations have been used with some success in such instances as:

a. Direct surface application to superficial basal cell lesions on the skin, especially 5 FU.

b. Direct injection infiltration of growths, e.g. subcutaneous secondary nodules of breast or lung cancer.

## Combination chemotherapy

Useful results came from agents used singly, but there was always an obvious possibility that a *combination* of two or more drugs might be superior to a single agent, just as several antibiotics together may be more potent in eradicating bacterial infection. One drug in the combination may kill tumour cells resistant to the other drugs. There will also be less opportunity for resistant cell lines to be left.

Another variation is to use them in *sequence – sequential therapy –* over a definite cycle. Examples:

Choriocarcinoma – p. 232.

Acute leukaemia – p. 236.

*Hodgkin's disease.* At first, single agents were used continuously for the late stages – mustine, vinca alkaloids (vincristine or vinblastine), procarbazine, and corticosteroids (prednisolone, etc). When one drug ceased to be effective, another was tried, in the above order. The results were certainly encouraging, with complete remission in 25 per cent and 25 per cent five-year survival. A major breakthrough was the introduction of *quadruple therapy,* four drugs used together – the now famous *MOPP regime* (M = mustine, O = oncovin = vincristine, P = procarbazine, P = prednisone). Complete remission now came in 80 per cent with 75 per cent five-year survival – a revolutionary achievement on any reckoning. *This regime is now the standard treatment* in all but the early stages of Hodgkin's and many non-Hodgkin's lymphomas. Minor variations are in use, e.g. some prefer vinblastine to vincristine (oncovin). One scheme is as follows:

Prednisolone 40 mg

Procarbazine 100 mg/m$^2$ daily for two weeks.

Vinblastine 10 mg on days 0, 7.

Mustine 6 mg/m$^2$ on days 0,7.

Note – m$^2$ = (per) square metre of body surface area. This is a better way of estimating dosage than body weight, especially in children. The body surface area is obtained from measurements of height and weight, with the aid of a nomogram (a diagrammatic mathematical device for getting a speedy result instead of having to make elaborate calculations). An average adult has a surface area bout 1.6 m$^2$.

Each course takes a fortnight. Patients need not be in hospital, except perhaps overnight, and on the first course, to observe reactions. After two weeks' rest the next course is begun. Courses are repeated at monthly intervals to a total of 6-10. If remission is complete, further courses are given at three-monthly intervals for a year, and at four-monthly intervals for the next year.

## The general principles of combination therapy are

1. The drugs should be effectual as single agents, but have different modes of action.

2. Treatment is pulsed – i.e. a short intensive course is followed by a free interval before the next. This gives time for recovery of bone marrow, bowel mucosa, nervous system and immune mechanisms. High doses given over short periods are generally better than low doses given over long periods.

3. Each drug should have a different major toxic effect, so that, while the therapeutic effect is cumulative, specific toxicity is minimised. Drugs of the same group, e.g. alkylating agents, should not usually be combined.

4. There is less chance of resistance to any one agent showing itself, since potentially resistant cells are likely to be vulnerable to one of the other agents.

5. Different drugs are believed to exert their effects at different points in the cell's developmental cycle, e.g. mustine acts at any stage of the cycle, whether the cell is resting or in mitosis (like radiation). Vinblastine, vincristine and methotrexate act in the phase of DNA synthesis, before mitosis. Cyclophosphamide, 5 FU and actinomycin-D are inactive in the resting stage, but active at any stage of the mitotic cycle. Combinations are therefore calculated to achieve a higher percentage kill.

There is now a long list of multiple drug regimes. Some will be mentioned under acute leukaemia (p. 236). Others in use include – COPAD (cyclophosphamide, oncovin, prednisone, adriamycin), VAC (vincristine, actinomycin-D, cyclophosphamide), MOB (methotrexate, oncovin, bleomycin) and many similar combinations. Experience is steadily accumulating and this is perhaps the most actively growing edge of the oncological attack. The shape of things to come is emerging from the shadows, but it will be many years before experience can be sifted to give us the most successful regimes.

## Combined radiotherapy and chemotherapy

This is another attractive possibility. Examples:

1. Acute lymphoblastic leukaemia in children, where results have been dramatically improved by irradiating the central nervous system (skull and spinal cord) after remission is achieved by drugs – see p. 182-3.

2. Ewing's tumour – it is always wise to assume that there is disseminated occult disease even if only one bone is clinically affected. Results are now markedly improving by irradiation of the bone first, then intermittent multi-drug therapy – see p. 187-8.

## Combined surgery and adjuvant chemotherapy

This is another obvious field to explore. Drugs are given after primary surgery, to destroy silent microscopic metastases and so increase the proportion of long-term survivors. So far, this combination has been applied mainly in children's tumours, with considerable success – e.g. Wilms's embryoma of kidney (see Ch. 14).

In theory this combination ought to be effective, and many attempts were made to improve results in the common adult cancers – lung, breast, etc. – using single agents, but with little or no success. Warning voices have been raised that such therapy might even be worse than useless, by depressing immunological defence mechanisms. With increased experience of combination therapy, the problems are now being tackled again. Promising examples are:

1. Bone cancer. Most cases (80 per cent) are doomed because of early silent secondaries before operation (p. 167). Recent adjuvant chemotherapy immediately after amputation has shown improved early results which will, we hope, be maintained with increased permanent salvage.

2. Breast cancer. Early spread is again the menace. Trials are now in progress using adjuvant chemotherapy in patients with proved axillary secondary nodes. It is a considerable burden on the patient to undergo such *long-term chemotherapy, which carries its own hazards*. But since we know that the presence of axillary secondaries lowers the five-year survival from 70 per cent to 30 per cent it *may* be worthwhile. We have the lessons learned from the disseminated lymphomas to guide us, and we know that useful improvement can often be obtained even in advanced breast cancer, from multi-drug therapy. The hope is that long-term freedom and normal life expectancy will be achieved. At the least, there should be a longer disease – free interval before recurrent trouble. Cautious trials for several years will be needed before we can tell whether the risks outweigh the benefits.

## Cancers cured by chemotherapy

It is now possible to talk of radical curative cytotoxic therapy, where drugs are the sole – or the chief – means of treatment. Some examples have already been given – acute leukaemia (p. 182) advanced Hodgkin's (p. 179). Two further examples will now be described, for their special interest and as signposts to future possibilities.

1. *Choriocarcinoma* (or Chorionepithelioma). This is the malignant variety of *gestational trophoblastic disease*. The fertilised ovum gives rise to the trophoblast which burrows into the endometrial wall to implant and nourish the ovum. Maternal tissue is destroyed till a balance is struck between fetal and maternal elements with eventual formation of the placenta. This equilibrium may be disturbed, by factors unknown, with production of disorders ranging from the simple to the highly malignant. It is unique among tumours, as it is derived not from tissues of the host, but from a 'parasite' (the fetus).

The simple variety is known as *hydatidiform mole,* where maternal tissue is invaded somewhat more than normally. The intensely malignant type is the *choriocarcinoma*. It is almost always a result of pregnancy, usually soon after, and half of them are preceded by moles. The uterus becomes enlarged, with ulceration and haemorrhage. Vaginal bleeding may be very heavy. Early, even the first, signs may come from secondaries, e.g. in lungs, with cough and dyspnoea. Diagnosis is confirmed by microscopy of fragments passed via the vagina or after uterine curettage.

*Hormone tests* are important. The tissue produces large amounts of *human chorionic gonadotrophia (HCG)* – the basis of pregnancy tests. This is very valuable both as an aid to diagnosis and to monitor progress after treatment, since persistently positive tests point to the presence of metastases.

*Treatment* used to be by hysterectomy and/or radiotherapy. Surgery is now rarely practised, and though the growth is radiosensitive, modern treatment now consists essentially of chemotherapy.

The most valuable drug is methotrexate in fairly high dosage, with folinic acid 'rescue'. Severe toxicity may result, and special isolation units are desirable (though not essential) to counter the complications. A good response is achieved in over 80 per cent. In refractory cases, combinations including 6-mercaptopurine and actinomycin-D may be successful.

If the growth is still confined to the uterus, the long-term success rate is 90 per cent, but if there are distant metastases, this drops to 25 per cent. After successful chemotherapy, further pregnancies are possible – though the high risk of gene mutations in the ovarian germ cells may make this a doubtful blessing.

This is a remarkable result by any standard, and represents perhaps the greatest triumph yet of chemotherapy in cancer. But choriocarcinoma is not a typical cancer. It arises in fetal tissue which is genetically 'foreign' to the host (the patient) and is therefore likely to give rise to antigens. Immunological factors almost certainly play a considerable part in the response, and this would account for the spontaneous regression (with no treatment at all) even of metastases, which certainly can occur on rare occasions – (see p. 23).

It does not follow therefore that other tumours will respond as well, on the basis of our present knowledge. Still, this does not lessen the immense practical value of the treatment, or its theoretical importance in pointing the way to potential similar triumphs in other lesions.

2. *Burkitt's tumour.* In 1958 a British surgeon, Burkitt, described a peculiar tumour affecting the upper and lower jaws and abdominal viscera in African children. Histologically it was a type of lymphoma, probably lymphosarcomatous; sporadic cases occur outside Africa – in Europe, USA, etc. Growth is very rapid, and without treatment most die within six months. Surgery is difficult, mutilating and usually ineffectual, since in clinical jaw cases there is usually undetected abdominal involvement also.

The treatment of choice is cytotoxic – methotrexate or cyclophosphamide – better still, both together. Severe marrow depression follows, the hair always falls out and cystitis is frequent. But complete regression occurs in over 50 per cent of cases, with apparent cure in 15 per cent. In case of recurrence, re-treatment may succeed.

There are also other intriguing aspects. The geographical area of distribution is exactly the same as that of disease – carrying insects, e.g. mosquitoes; a virus is now believed to be the causative agent. Just as with choriocarcinoma, immunological factors probably play a part – even a predominant part – in the success of treatment. Complete regression can occur after even a single dose of the drug – as though some mechanism had been triggered into action. Even spontaneous remissions are known to happen. Clearly, it is a very untypical cancer, but at least an interesting and exciting pointer to possibilities of wider application in other cancers.

**Summary conclusion**

Cytotoxic chemotherapy is a recent and revolutionary development and has a long way still to go. In the last edition of this book, only a few years ago, we said 'We cannot yet claim any permanently curative results' – but the situation has already changed. Experience was inevitably slow in accumulating, mistakes were made, toxicity was alarming, the use of single agents was the rule, and initial optimism was succeeded by a wave of pessimism. This is a common sequence of events when new modes of treatment are discovered – just as in the case of ionising radiation.

So far, the greatest successes have been in the field of the disseminated 'soft' tumours – such as leukaemias and lymphomas. In children's tumours, the impact has also been revolutionary. In the common adult 'solid' cancers, the contribution has so far been disappointing, but the field is being worked over again, in the light of our newer knowledge of combination therapy and a more scientific appreciation of what is called 'cell population kinetics' as a basis for correct dosage, timing etc. The role of pre-operative and post-operative chemotherapy, and the optimum combinations of surgery, radiation and drugs for each particular type of cancer – not forgetting the potential critical importance of immunology – have still to be worked out. We are really only at the beginning of the road.

The brilliant results, e.g. in choriocarcinoma and Burkitt's tumour give us inspiration and hope. The recent spectacular advances in molecular biology, a knowledge of the key biochemical structures of the cell, especially the nucleus and mitosis, could well enable us, before the end of the century, to pin-point the initial steps in malignancy. If so, we could – one hopes – devise rational means of either forestalling or correcting it.

# 14. Cancer in Children

*Alas, that Spring should vanish with the Rose!*
*That Youth's sweet-scented Manuscript should close!*
Edward Fitzgerald (Omar Khayyam)

Between the ages of one and fifteen – after accidents, poisoning and violence – *malignant disease is the commonest cause of death in Britain.* This is due to the control of infectious childhood diseases in the past quarter century (diphtheria, whooping cough, meningitis, measles, etc. etc.). In the past decade or so there have been major advances in treatment and prognosis of several types of malignancy. Since the total number of cases is relatively small, it is best for treatment to be concentrated in a few special centres, where a specialist team can handle all the cases from a wide region and so accumulate expertise for the benefit of all patients – otherwise nobody would gain sufficient experience to be really competent. The team should include – paediatric physician, surgeon, radiotherapist, chemotherapist and/or haematologist.

To keep matters in perspective – a general practitioner is unlikely to see more than a couple of cases in a working lifetime. Diagnosis is in any case usually difficult, since the early signs tend to be vague – failure to thrive, fever, pallor, loss of appetite, headache – all of which are common to many other disorders.

In most types, the mode of origin of the growth differs from that in adults, being a developmental malformation (which may even be present at birth) rather than a result of 'chronic irritation'. Hence surface (epithelial) tissues, which are the usual sufferers from repeated trauma, are not the usual sites of origin in children.

Hereditary and genetic factors play a part. This is very obvious in retinoblastoma. Other congenital defects are liable to be associated, e.g. mongols have 30 times the normal risk of developing leukaemia.

Immunological factors are also probably important. The antibody recognition and defence systems are immature in the young child, and this may account for the frequency of acute lymphoblastic leukaemia. Whether virus infection plays any part in induction is still uncertain and unproved, though the idea is very tempting, especially as comparable leukaemias can certainly be induced by viruses in laboratory animals.

Just as normal growth in children is more pronounced than in adults, so malignant growth tends to be rapid and throw off early metastases.

They are correspondingly *radiosensitive,* but this unfortunately does not mean radiocurable.

*Types.* The commonest cancers are:

| | |
|---|---:|
| Leukaemia – mainly acute | 35 per cent |
| Central nervous system – glioma | 30 per cent |
| Connective tissues – including bone | 12 per cent |
| Neuroblastoma | 8 per cent |
| Wilms's tumour – nephroblastoma | 5 per cent |

**Acute leukaemia**

This is the commonest cancer of all. It is of lymphocytic (lymphoblastic) type in 80-90 per cent. The clinical picture comprises fever, headache, ulceration of mucosal surfaces (mouth etc.), purpuric haemorrhages, loss of weight and maybe prostration. There may be enlarged lymph nodes, spleen and liver.

Until 1948, only supportive therapy was possible – blood transfusion for anaemia, antibiotics for infection, drugs for pain; and few cases survived more than a few months. Cytotoxic drugs have now brought remarkable improvement, and the rapid progress over the last three decades has seen the prognosis change from death within a few weeks of diagnosis to an odds-on chance of five years disease-free survival and presumed cure.

Neither surgery nor radiation is of any value. In addition to general supportive therapy, the mainstay of treatment is chemotherapy, with various combinations of drugs.

The basis of therapy is the simple concept of preventing cell division by drug interference, and more progress has been made latterly by applying available drugs in different ways than by the introduction of new agents.

Therapy is seen as falling into three parts, these being *Remission Induction, Cytoreduction, and Remission Maintenance.*

*Remission Induction,* i.e. removal of all detectable signs of the disease, is easily achieved in the majority of cases by three once weekly intravenous injections of Vincristine at a dose of 1 to 1.5 mg per square metre, coupled with three weeks continuous therapy of Prednisolone at 40 mg per square metre per day.

At this stage advantage is taken of the patient's improved condition to *consolidate the situation* with other, some more aggressive, agents including Adriamycin, Cyclophosphamide and Asparaginase. The brain and meninges are treated by cranial irradiation and intrathecal Methotrexate at this time (see p. 183), as the drugs given are inefficient at crossing the blood-brain barrier. (Leukaemia recurrence in these sites was a common problem before this precautionary therapy).

*Remission is then maintained* for a period of *two to three years by* the cyclical application of several agents, usually including mercaptopurine, methotrexate, prednisolone and further occasional vincristine. After this time the treatment is stopped, as it is thought that the risks from the dangers of continued therapy outweigh the diminishing risk of leukaemic relapse.

Protocols for therapy of this condition differ in detail, and cases with features suggesting a poor prognosis (a greater leukaemic cell mass at diagnosis, patients older than 14 years, those with mediastinal tumours and negro children) are often treated more aggressively at the start. Immunotherapy, the idea of stimulating the patient's own immune response to kill a (presumed) remaining few leukaemic cells after chemotherapy, has not found a regular place yet in the management of acute lymphoblastic leukaemias. Much research into improving therapy, of course, continues.

An important adjunct to primary therapy discussed above is the secondary supportive therapy. This would include the facilities of a special centre with much experience of acute leukaemia, and the availability of staff and materials to cope with the two chief consequences of disease or therapeutically induced bone marrow failure; haemorrhage and infection.

Platelet-rich blood fractions to treat bleeding through lack of platelets are available readily now at all major blood transfusion centres, but leucocyte transfusions to aid antibiotic therapy of the septicaemias easily acquired by leukaemic patients with marrow failure are still only available in a few centres. This is due to the technical problems of collection and storage.

Such supportive measures have dramatically reduced mortality early in the course of leukaemia therapy, and the increasing tendency to centralize care of these patients may do so further.

For pain in the limbs due to local bone deposits, small doses of X-rays – a few hundred rads – are valuable. Neurological complications used to be fairly common, due to meningeal deposits, with increased intracranial pressure, headache, vomiting and papilloedema. Prophylactic treatment as described on p. 183 has largely eliminated this.

The *psychological handling* of parents and child is important. Parents should be told the whole truth from the start – that cure may not be possible, but treatment will relieve symptoms and allow the child to lead a nearly normal life for a variable length of time, though with necessary intervals for treatment in hospital.

*Results* of intensive chemotherapy have been a steady increase in length of survival. *Remissions occur in almost all cases – 95 per cent.* There are now scores of patients who have survived over five years, and some more than ten, so that we can look forward to at least a proportion of permanent 'cures'.

*Acute leukaemia in adults* is treated by the same principal drugs, with minor variations in technique.

**Intracranial tumours** (see also Ch. 9)

These are mainly: astrocytoma, medulloblastoma and ependymoma.

a. *Astrocytoma* is treated surgically and complete removal may occasionally be possible. If not, radiation should be added and the prognosis, though poor, is not hopeless.

b. *Medulloblastoma* is treated by preliminary surgery to relieve obstruction, followed by radiotherapy – described on p. 152. Useful results are obtainable, as the growth is very radiosensitive. Cytotoxic therapy with vincristine and CCNU has recently been found to be a useful adjuvant for primary treatment or recurrence.

c. *Ependymoma* is treated on the same lines as astrocytoma.

**Wilms's tumour of kidney**

This is also called Wilms's *Embryoma,* or *Nephroblastoma,* described by Max Wilms (1867-1918), professor of surgery at Heidelberg, Germany. It presents between the ages of a few months and about eight years – average five years – usually as a mass causing abdominal enlargement. Intravenous pyelography helps to confirm the diagnosis. Early regional node and lung secondaries are common. Treatment includes surgery, radiation and chemotherapy.

Full pre-treatment assessment should be made including chest film and skeletal survey (isotope whole body scan if available).

*Treatment.* Till recently, the standard treatment was immediate surgical nephrectomy plus post-operative radiation. Sometimes pre-operative radiation was practised if the mass was very large, in order to shrink it and improve the surgeon's chance. The results were poor, since more than 50 per cent proved to have silent lung metastases at the time, which were ultimately fatal. Improvement came only when cytotoxic chemotherapy was added to supplement surgery and radiation, to control these latent metastases, and when cases were concentrated and managed at specialist centres.

At operation, the surgeon removes the kidney with its associated vessels and nodes. If nodes appear to be involved, he also carries out a block dissection of paraortic nodes on the affected side, from the diaphragm above to the bifurcation of the aorta below. He examines the abdomen for malignant spread – liver, bowel, pelvis, etc. It is very helpful if he outlines the limits of the tumour bed by radio-opaque clips for the guidance of the radiotherapist in laying out the radiation fields.

*Radiation technique.* Radiation is begun as soon as possible, and in children it is not necessary to await wound healing. Cobalt beam or megavoltage should be used. A pair of parallel fields, antero-posterior, covers the tumour bed and regional nodes. They extend from the dome of the diaphragm to the sacral promontory, and cross the midline to include the whole width of the vertebrae. The other kidney is carefully shielded with the aid of the IVP films. The typical dosage is 3250 rads in four weeks.

An alternative technique, if there is evidence of spread, is an abdominal 'bath', treating the whole of the peritoneal cavity, from pelvic floor to diaphragm. The femoral heads are shielded, so as not to interfere with bone growth. The opposite kidney is shielded from the start − any involvement here is left to be dealt with by the subsequent chemotherapy. A depth dose of 3000 rads is given in five weeks.

Pulmonary secondaries should be treated by chest baths, irradiating all the lung tissue. The shoulder joints are excluded. A tumour dose of 2000 rads is given in three weeks. Even if lung secondaries appear localised, it is unsafe to treat less than the whole chest.

*Radiation reactions* must be watched − nausea, vomiting, white cell and platelet falls. The dosage and overall time may need adjustment accordingly. Impairment of growth of the vertebrae may result in slight but insignificant shortening of height. Formerly, when the border of the treatment field was taken only up to the midline, only half of any vertebral body was affected; this could lead to unbalanced growth and distortion, with resultant scoliosis. If the whole vertebral width is included, as it should be, this inequality of bone growth is avoided; but scoliosis can still occur from fibrosis and contracture of the muscles of the back on the treated side, especially if additional supplementary dosage is given (as some advise) to the tumour bed locally.

If abdominal baths are applied in girls, amenorrhoea and sterility will follow. This should be explained to the family.

*Cytotoxic chemotherapy.* The chief purpose of *adjuvant cytotoxic therapy* is to destroy silent secondaries in their microscopic stage. There are various good regimes, and treatment can even begin on the day of operation. One regime is vincristine (intravenous) once a week for six doses, then once a fortnight for the next two years. It has little effect on bone marrow, but the chief toxic effects are on the nervous system − see p. 226.

Another good drug is actinomycin-D. Adriamycin is now also under trial. Agents have usually been given singly, one or the other. The latest evidence goes to show that their effect is even better when combined; a multi-drug regime will almost certainly be the rule in future.

*Prognosis.* Younger children tend to do better than older, but this is because the older child tends to have the more advanced lesion. Formerly, the average five-year survival was about 30 per cent and about 50 per cent for children under two. Now, at the best specialist centres, rates of 80 to 90 per cent are being achieved, giving Wilms's tumour a better prognosis than any other childhood cancer.

## Neuroblastoma

This is the commonest solid tumour in children. It is rare in adults, and the great majority occur before the age of five; over half are under two years, or it may even be present at birth.

*Pathology.* It arises in sympathetic nervous tissue, which includes the medulla of the adrenal gland and similar tissue at other sites (posterior abdomen, mediastinum, pelvis, neck). There is considerable variation in its biological behaviour. In a few rare cases, mostly under one year old, spontaneous regression occurs, with maturation into an adult non-malignant form – even if disease is advanced and metastatic – but most spread locally and soon metastasise. *Most cases already have widespread secondaries when first seen.*

Local spread is to kidney, liver etc. Lymphatic spread is to paraortic nodes. Blood spread takes it to liver and bones; but rarely to lungs, in contrast with Wilms's tumour.

*Clinical features.* There may be a painless swelling in abdomen or loin, but often the first indication is due to metastases, e.g. bone pain or pathological fracture. Widespread bone secondaries with an occult primary is a common picture. The liver may be palpably enlarged. Skull metastases may cause unilateral exophthalmos (protrusion of the eye). Intravenous pyelography (IVP) helps to distinguish it from Wilms's tumour, by showing it to be extrarenal. A full radiographic skeletal survey should be made, and bone marrow examined for malignant involvement. A total body isotope bone scan is better than radiography for revealing secondaries.

*Catecholamines.* The physiological activity of the sympathetic nervous system is mediated by complex organic substances called catecholamines. Metabolic breakdown products appear in the blood and are excreted in the urine. Most cases of neuroblastoma excrete abnormally large quantities, and the most important product is called vanillyl – mandelic acid (VMA). Biochemical tests of urine are very valuable both for diagnosis and to monitor progress under treatment and detect early recurrence.

*Treatment.* Surgery, radiation and chemotherapy all have important roles. Since most cases are generalised at the time of diagnosis, generalised (systemic) treatment is indicated in all but the early stages of development. Complete *surgical excision* is rarely possible, because of extensive local infiltration, but partial excision may be possible. Surgery therefore is seldom the main form of treatment.

*Post-operative radiation* is usually advisable. In abdominal cases (i.e. the majority), it will be necessary to include one or both kidneys, but the kidney dosage should not exceed 1500 rads in two weeks. Technique and dosage are similar to that for Wilms's tumour (see above). For an abdominal case, not more than 2500 rads should be given in 4 weeks, by a megavoltage pair depending on the age and the treatment volume. It may be impossible to avoid irradiating the ovaries. In thoracic or pelvic cases, smaller volumes are involved, and 2500 to 3000 rads may be given in 3 to 4 weeks; humeral or femoral epiphyses are shielded.

Radiation is good palliation for painful bone deposits – single doses of 750 to 1000 rads suffice.

For inoperable tumours, some use radiation in the hope of causing shrinkage and possibly making the mass operable. It is better to start with chemotherapy, and if shrinkage occurs, then proceed to surgery, maybe with the help of pre-operative radiation.

*Cytotoxic therapy* plays a major role and is finding increasing application now. It is the best initial treatment for widespread metastatic disease, and the initial response is usually good, with pain relief and bone healing. Unfortunately it has not so far reduced the recurrence rate. The best drugs are – vincristine, cyclophosphamide and adriamycin together, intravenously, at fortnightly intervals. This can be done on an out-patient basis. They cause some sickness, for which an anti-emetic drug should be given, and also total alopecia (baldness). The parents should be warned of this, and wigs provided for all but the youngest patients. The hair always grows again. Treatment should be continued at weekly or fortnightly intervals for up to two years.

Neuroblastoma is remarkable in that even cases with very widespread metastasis, liver, bone, etc., are not hopeless, and are worth treating. The response to cytotoxics may be astonishingly good.

*Prognosis.* Neuroblastoma shows the highest rate of spontaneous regression of any tumour – up to 8 per cent. Survival depends more on the child's age than the extent of disease. Survival for two years usually means cure. For children below one year old, the two-year survival is 75 per cent; over one year, it drops to 20 per cent. Even with minimal treatment, response in the very young is so good, that there must be immunological factors at work to account for it; these factors are lost as the child ages. The outlook is particularly bad in the presence of bone involvement, except in the very young.

In practice, the response is poor in most cases. Intensive combined therapy has not much improved the survival rate (in contrast to Wilms's tumour and rhabdomyosarcoma). Palliation can usually be achieved, but overall survival has not changed.

*Bone tumours* are relatively common between the ages of 5 and 25. They include osteosarcoma, chondrosarcoma and reticulum cell sarcoma; also the dubious entity called Ewing's sarcoma. Their management is described on pp. 167-9, 187-8.

*Soft tissue sarcomas* include fat (liposarcoma), muscle (myosarcoma) and connective tissue (fibrosarcoma), and may appear any time after birth.

## Rhabdomyosarcoma

This is the commonest of all the childhood soft tissue sarcomas. It occurs at two main sites – (a) head and neck, including orbit – 80 per cent and (b) lower urinary tract. It is highly malignant, grows rapidly, invades locally and spreads widely via lymph and blood.

Primary treatment is usually by *surgery,* but even radical removal often fails, because of local recurrence or distant metastasis. Post--operative *radiation* should be given — 5000 rads in four weeks if possible.

Till recently, long-term survival was rare, but intensive *chemotherapy* is now improving the prognosis considerably. Surgery and postoperative radiation are used, plus a regime of triple chemotherapy using vincristine, actinomycin-D and cyclophosphamide in regular pulses. This begins immediately on diagnosis, continues throughout the course of radiation, and carries on for two years. Adriamycin is now also in use.

Complete regression is now achieved in most cases, and mutilating surgery is no longer justifiable. It is too early to assess the long-term prognosis with the new regime, but current results are very encouraging.

### Retinoblastoma

This is a rare tumour, but of great 'interest as one of the very few hereditary growths, and the only genetically determined neoplasm that is malignant from the start. It is caused by a gene mutation which is dominant, so that parents who have been cured of retinoblastoma are very likely to find the disease in their children. Most cases, however, appear in children with no such family history, i.e. as a result of new spontaneous mutations.

It arises from primitive retinal cells, and forms flat or projecting masses which invade the retina and other tissues of the eye, eventually destroying vision and in extreme cases invading orbital soft tissue, bone etc. The chief route of spread is along the optic nerve, to the cranial cavity and brain. Distant metastasis is late, to nodes, lungs etc.

*Clinical features.* Most cases are unexpected, and discovered by the parents at an average age of two, rarely after six. There may be a squint, or an opaque light reflex ('cat's eye reflex') in the normally dark pupil, followed by loss of vision. These cases are always locally advanced. In 25 to 30 per cent of cases growths are bilateral, and the other eye should be examined ophthalmoscopically at regular intervals after the first eye has been treated, to detect new lesions at an early stage. If there is a family history of retinoblastoma, all children should be examined from infancy regularly, up to the age of five.

*Treatment.* For the typical new (i.e. advanced) case, there is no hope of useful vision, even though the growth is radiosensitive, and the eye should be removed surgically. As great a length as possible of the optic nerve is removed with the eye, and carefully examined microscopically. If the nerve is found to be invaded up to the cut end, there will be clearly be residual tumour in the remaining part, and postoperative radiation should be given to the orbit and the region of the nerve stump. A cobalt beam wedge pair is suitable, giving 4500 rads in four weeks.

The situation is very different with a small growth discovered in the other eye, or in a child examined because of the family history. Here every effort should be made to preserve not merely the eye, but also useful vision. Radiation is here the treatment of choice, since the growth is radiosensitive. The most favourable situation is the posterior part of the retina, for the anterior part with the lens can then be spared. One technique is external radiation by a single lateral megavoltage field carefully aimed behind the lens, and directed 5° posteriorly to avoid the opposite eye. A tumour dose of the same order as above is given. Immobilisation of young children may be a problem; it may be necessary to give a soporific to put the child to sleep. If so, treatment is preferably three times a week instead of the usual five, and 10 to 15 per cent must be deducted from the total dosage to compensate for the larger fractions in the same overall time.

Another technique is shown in Fig. 14.1. The external surface of the eyeball is exposed surgically, and a specially prepared disc holding radioactive cobalt is sutured in position, overlying the tumour mass. The exact position of the growth must be determined by previous ophthalmoscopy. The disc is removed at a second operation about a week later. There is a range of applicators, circular, semicircular and crescentic, made of platinum loaded with cobalt. They are calibrated to give a minimum tumour dose of 4000 rads; the highest dose, at the surface of the eyeball will be over 20 000 rads, but this is well tolerated. This can be very satisfactory treatment for a small solitary lesion, but since growths are commonly multicentric i.e. more than one in the same eye, external radiation is more widely applicable.

*Prognosis.* For a rare tumour like this, and the need for specialised and meticulous technique, it is advisable for treatment to be concentrated at a very few centres in any country, so that adequate experience can be gained. Prognosis depends very much on the stage of advancement at the time of treatment. The aim of any treatment except surgery is preservation of useful vision – otherwise surgery would always be the method of choice. Post-operative radiation for known residues is certainly useful. Most small tumours at the back of the eye can be controlled with useful vision – up to 90 per cent. This falls to 30 per cent for multiple growths or in the anterior part of the eye.

*Burkitt's tumour* is another fascinating lesion – see pp. 233-4.

*Benign tumours* are worth a mention. The commonest is the ordinary *angiomatous skin birthmark,* which generally needs no treatment (see p. 246). However, benign haemangioma may involve subcutaneous tissue, viscera or bone, and can even be fatal owing to haemorrhage, pressure and obstruction. Troublesome tumours should be excised if possible, as the response to radiation is not usually good enough. If excision is impracticable or dangerous, radiation is indicated.

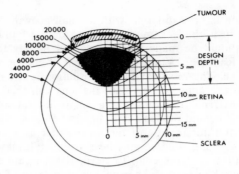

Fig. 14.1 A Colbalt-60 ophthalmic applicator in position at the back of the eye for treatment of a retinoblastoma (shown black). (Courtesy of the Radiochemical Centre, Amersham, England)

### Summary conclusion

Cancer in children is almost a speciality on its own. Since the total number of patients in any region is not large, treatment is best concentrated at special centres. Long-term results in the majority of cases are disappointing, and the nursing problems often formidable. Surgery, radiation and chemotherapy are all valuable, especially in combination, and recent results show worthwhile improvement in most types of tumour. Cures are certainly obtainable, especially in the younger patients.

# 15. Radiotherapy in Non-malignant Disorders

*They say miracles are past.*
Shakespeare (All's Well That Ends Well)

Cancer is not the only disease process where radiation can be useful. It was inevitable that such a powerful weapon should be widely explored and applied in the early days, before its dangers and limitations were – or could be – realised. There is, in fact, scarcely a disorder in the textbooks for which radiotherapy has not been tried by some enthusiast in the pioneer days, and unfortunately a good deal of damage – even fatal damage – was done unwittingly before the serious consequences emerged.

A striking example came to light only a few years ago. Radiation of an enlarged thymus in infancy used to be practised, and it caused gratifying shrinkage. Years later, however, carcinoma of the thyroid developed in some cases, undoubtedly induced by the effects of the rays on the immature thyroid cells.

Where treatment appeared to be useful, e.g. in many skin disorders, repeated dosage was commonly given for recurrent trouble, since the cumulative effects even of low doses were for long not appreciated.

Nowadays the field for non-malignant treatment has been severely restricted, both because of accumulated knowledge of the long-term effects on the various organs and the development of modern specific therapy such as antibiotics.

*Mode of action.* This is not fully understood, but the following mechanisms are probably at work:

1. In *inflammatory conditions* – breakdown of white blood cells and liberation of enzymes and antibodies; suppression of immune reactions (lymphocytes); promotion of more rapid 'ageing' of inflammatory cells, thereby accelerating the healing process.

2. *Reduction of excessive secretion* from glands – endocrine (thyroid, ovary, pituitary), sebaceous and sweat glands of skin.

3. *Reduction of cellular infiltration,* e.g. in eczema.

4. *Epilation* – destruction of hair follicles.

5. *Anti-pruritic* – the mode of action is quite obscure.

6. *Reduction of benign overgrowth,* e.g. keloids, warts, angioma, hyperkeratosis.

We will outline the chief situations where radiation may still be of value.

## Dermatology

Twenty five years ago it was possible to say that X-rays were the most important therapeutic weapon of the dermatologist. With the advent of antibiotics, steroids, etc., this is no longer true, but radiation is still useful and large skin departments commonly have their own X-ray machines; otherwise their patients are treated in the radiotherapy department.

Since great penetration is not required – and would in fact be a positive drawback – low-voltage superficial X-ray units are used. These are described on p. 59. The most superficial type of all – *Grenz-ray* units – are particularly useful, since the very low penetration of Grenz rays gives them some notable advantages:

The epidermis can be treated with very little effect on deeper structures such as hair roots and sweat glands. It is difficult to cause serious skin damage, and late cancer production is unknown. There is no danger to underlying eyes, testes, bone etc., no risk of epilation, and treatments can be repeated many times.

When X-ray treatment is used in skin disorders, it is almost always as *a last resort, when other treatments have failed*. It is of value in:

a. *Chronic eczema* – especially hands and forearms.

b. *Acne vulgaris.*

c. *Acne rosacea.*

d. *Psoriasis* – especially palms and soles, and the nail bed. In this particular type, X-rays may be the treatment of choice.

e. *Pruritus ani.*

In all the above lesions, dosage is quite low – 50-100 rads – at weekly, fortnightly or monthly intervals. Accurate records must be kept, since relapses are common. *It is a good rule never to exceed a total of 1000 rads at any site during a patient's lifetime.*

f. *Epilation.* X-rays were once widely used for removing scalp hair in ringworm; also the beard in sycosis barbae. Antibiotics have now outmoded this. X-rays should never be used for cosmetic removal of unsightly hairs, since adequate dosage always risks skin atrophy.

The epilation effect is still of value in two conditions:

1. Inverted eyelashes.

2. Pilonidal sinus after local excision.

Doses about 1000 rads are needed, in a single shot.

g. *Angioma.* The common *strawberry naevus* – a birthmark of infants – may grow rapidly and alarmingly for weeks. Almost all regress spontaneously within a few years and the *best policy is masterful inactivity*. The few indications for active treatment are: (a) medical if it is causing trouble, such as feeding difficulty or respiratory obstruction, or threatens to ulcerate, and (b) psychological – to appease a worried mother who will not be reassured unless 'something is done'.

Possible treatments include – surgery, injection of coagulant chemicals, electro-coagulation, and freezing; or radiation, which is the simplest to apply. The speed of resolution can certainly be accelerated by treatment, and if the angioma is seen before its growth has reached its peak (which is not usually the case), a dose of superficial X-rays can be given, 400 rads. Care must be taken not to irradiate the gonads, epiphyses of bone, or the thyroid; if these are nearby, non-radiation methods are preferable.

*Port-wine stains* (capillary angioma) differ in not disappearing spontaneously and being usually unresponsive to X-rays, though improvement can sometimes be obtained by Grenz rays.

h. *Keloid* scars are unsightly and may itch and be painful. Cortisone injections may be helpful. Radiation, with doses of 1000 rads, can flatten an early vascular fleshy mass before thickening sets in, but not after it has fibrosed. An old keloid can be excised, and the line of excision irradiated to prevent recurrence. The same warnings about the proximity of the immature thyroid and gonads should be remembered, and radiation to the neck or pelvis is always best avoided in young people. Moreover, spontaneous regression is quite common.

i. *Warts,* especially plantar, used to be very commonly treated with X-rays, which are effective in single doses of 1000-1500 rads. However, necrosis has followed in too many cases – even though the proportion is very low indeed – and radiation is not to be recommended.

j. *Hyperkeratosis* will respond to adequate dosage – e.g. 2,000 rads (single shot) to a tiny nodule.

### Endocrine disorders

The excessive secretion of an overactive gland can always be repressed by adequate radiation, and this is of practical value in the following:
*1. Thyroid.* Hyperthyroidism (thyrotoxicosis) can be effectively controlled by radioactive iodine, which is often the method of choice. This technique is described on p. 193.
*2. Pituitary* (see also p. 152). In eosinophil adenoma, radiation usually relieves the pressure symptoms, but the hormonal effects (acromegaly) rarely improve. In basophil adenoma, the tumour is usually microscopic, and commonly associated with an adrenal tumour. If there is no demonstrable adrenal tumour, radiation may be given to the pituitary, since it is simple and carries no operative risk. In case of failure, surgery is still available.
*3. Ovary.* Excessive oestrogen secretion causes *menorrhagia,* and ovarian radiation is an effective alternative to hysterectomy. Radiation can be applied in two ways:
a. *Internal* – an intra-uterine radium tube, as used in treatment of uterine cancer, will irradiate and inhibit both the endometrium and the ovaries. A 50-mg tube is left in for 40-48 hr. General anaesthesia in hospital is needed and this provides the essential opportunity for a thorough pelvic examination, curettage and biopsy, to exclude malignan-

cy as the cause of bleeding. This technique is very effective and still used, though it can lead to some degree of endometritis and uterine discharge.

b. *External* — by megavoltage X-rays. A single dose usually suffices, but two or three treatments may be preferred, to avoid radiation sickness. *Note* — induction of an artificial menopause in this way involves *sterilisation* of the patient. In almost all cases, this raises no problems and is in fact desirable. It is wise, however, to obtain the written consent of both the patient and (if possible) her husband, who should be asked to sign a form stating that the effects of the treatment have been explained, understood and accepted.

## Rheumatic disorders

This is a mixed group of obscure pathology, and therapy of any kind is very often unsatisfactory. X-rays were once used extensively, but have now been largely given up. The following may still be considered:

*1. Ankylosing spondylitis.* This is a disabling process, mostly in young men, with pain and stiffness, leading to 'poker back' rigidity. Until 1955, deep X-ray therapy was widely and successfully used as the mainstay of treatment, directed either to the sacro-iliac joints alone, where the disease generally first appears, or the whole spine. Then it was discovered that a small proportion of treated patients developed leukaemia, undoubtedly as a late radiation effect and comparable to the leukaemia induced by atomic radiation from bombs, etc. (p. 14).

This led to abandonment of the treatment by most radiotherapists. But there are still a few cases where, if other methods fail, localised X-ray therapy can be quite justified for relief of a painful and crippling disorder. The slight risk (one in several thousand) should be fully explained to the patient, and the final choice left to him — more often than not, he will consider it an acceptable hazard.

*2. Osteo-arthritis,* especially of the knee joint, is difficult to relieve. X-rays can be helpful, and one or two short courses — but no more — can be justified.

*3. Capsulitis of the shoulder* (subacromial bursitis). Similar considerations apply here.

## Ophthalmology

The principal use now is for corneal lesions, especially vascularisation — described on p. 203-4.

## Peptic ulcers

The symptoms of gastric and duodenal ulcers are relieved by counteracting or abolishing the acid secreted by the gastric mucosa. Treatment is by medical and/or surgical measures. If conservative treatment fails and if surgery is contra-indicated by age, etc., radiation to inhibit or reduce acid secretion is worth a trial.

The technique is simple. The stomach is localised with a barium swallow and antero-posterior fields outlined. A megavoltage course of 1500 rads is given in 10 daily fractions.

## Miscellaneous

Other applications are mostly of historical interest only, with the inevitable record of undesirable or serious after-effects, such as permanent baldness after ringworm treatment, or osteosarcoma after treatment of bone tuberculosis.

# 16. Terminal Care and the Management of Pain

*And when we're worn,*
*Hack'd, hewn with constant service, thrown aside*
*To rust in peace, or rot in hospitals...*
                    Thomas Southerne (1660-1740)

## After-care

During and after a course of treatment, the patient should always be told what to expect by way of reactions and symptoms (e.g. alopecia). Explanations should always be given of what is being done, within his understanding. Reasons for special precautions with radium, radioactive iodine etc. should be outlined. This avoids alarm and promotes confidence.

Ward nurses should be in liaison with the radiographers in the treatment department, concerning such details as length of treatment, and skin and mucosal reactions.

On discharge from hospital, arrangements for attendance at follow-up clinics should be made, and the importance of supervision should be indicated, not so as to cause alarm, but to stress the value of the occasional check-up and to forestall further trouble. Appropriate arrangements for transport should be made if required.

The patient's home conditions are of prime importance. This aspect is apt to be overlooked by the doctor. For example, patients are sometimes allowed home at weekends during a prolonged course of treatment, even though home conditions may be quite unsuitable, e.g. he may live alone – and expose the patient to infection, undernourishment and dehydration. Ward sisters should enquire about this and be in active liaison with the medical social worker over all relevant matters. Financial and other help may be required, and the social services have an important part to play. Home helps and district nurses may be needed, and various agencies are available for assistance in many ways. They include – National Society for Cancer Relief, Marie Curie Cancer Foundation, British Legion, W.R.V.S., and local voluntary organisations, in addition to Social Security. Provision can be made for extra nourishment, heating, bedding, appliances, commode etc.

## What to tell

The problem generally arises of what to tell the patient and relatives about diagnosis and prognosis. The decision rests with the doctor in charge, but the nurses should be informed, so that they are aware of the situation and can act accordingly. Sometimes there is little or no difficulty; the patient is blissfully unaware – or appears so – and asks no questions. Often, however, he is openly or secretly worried and may try to extract information from the nurses. Contact with the patient will often reveal to the nurse how much he knows – or suspects or fears – and this knowledge should be passed on to the doctor, so that doctor and nurse can work together and follow the line considered to be in the particular patient's best interest. It is sometimes appropriate to say, e.g. 'It's an ulcer that needs treatment to heal it before it can develop into a cancer'. At other times the patient may show himself fully aware of the diagnosis, and it may often be possible to assure him that the outlook in his case is very favourable, and that there are many patients well cured of the same disease as his. Even if we think it inappropriate to speak of 'cure' in a particular case, it is usually helpful to point out that many cancers can be successfully controlled for long periods of time, like pernicious anaemia and diabetes, and the patient can lead a normal life.

In any event, it is nearly always advisable to inform at least one responsible member of the family of the situation and prospects. This is not always a simple matter, e.g. a spouse may be emotionally unstable and unable to 'take it' – and to tell him or her may be a mistaken kindness. The family doctor should be consulted in case of doubt.

The problem naturally becomes more acute if curative treatment fails or is ruled out from the start, and in most terminal cases. No general rule can be laid down – each case must be treated individually, and we must learn to 'play it by ear', trying to do what seems best for the individual. There is, of course, room for differences of opinion here, ranging from 'never tell a lie' to 'Never tell the whole truth'. We have already discussed some aspects of this problem (pp. 39-41). Some patients will simply not believe the truth if told bluntly – they reject it emotionally. We must distinguish between the demand for 'the truth' and the desire for reassurance (e.g. 'Is it very serious, doctor?'). Fortunately, in most cases it is quite easy to do so, and so spare the patient the worst.

In a few cases – not very common – a patient really wants the truth and is entitled to know it, particularly if he has important financial and family affairs to arrange (though even here both patient and doctor may come to regret it). All one can say is that it is seldom if ever pardonable to rob any patient of his sole remaining resource, i.e. hope, even at a late stage. The novelist Balzac said 'Hope is a thin diet, but very stimulating'. Florence Nightingale is alleged to have called it the greatest impertinence to tell a dying patient he would not recover and destroy all hope for the future. It is impossible to judge precisely what effect it will have on a given patient – even the most stoical and well-balanced – to be told he is approaching death. Often enough, the patient knows he is dying (and the doctor or nurse knows that he knows) – but it is the last thing he wants to be told. There is a mutual conspiracy of silence — a dignified and civilised silence, each side wishing to spare the other. It is usually better so.

## Pain and its management

In physical and medical care, relief of pain is by far the most important aspect. Fortunately nowadays we can virtually always relieve it, often almost completely, or at least make it tolerable. In terminal malignancy pain tends to be constant, and the guiding principle should be *constant control* — a schedule to *anticipate pain rather than 'treat' it*. There must be no clock-watching, no waiting anxiously for the next dose, no need to have to feel the pain in order to justify a tablet or injection. It is easy to forget that the malignancy may not be the source of the pain. The possibility of constipation, bedsores, cystitis, peptic ulcer, arthritis etc. should be remembered.

Large doses of powerful drugs are very rarely necessary. *Small but frequent regular doses* suffice, and will obviate the need for really large doses. In this way we can generally master what is almost worse than pain itself — i.e. the fear of pain, which is the cause of so much distress.

*Analgesics.* The drugs available are legion. But it is best to get to know a few only, acquire experience of them, and use them skilfully.

For *mild pain,* the following may be used every 4-6 hr:

Aspirin — 2-4 tablets (300 mg each) better as soluble aspirin (Aspirin soluble tablets B.P. — 300 mg) or as 'Nu-Seals', enteric coated containing 325 mg aspirin B.P., to avoid gastric irritation.

Paracetamol (Panadol) 2 tablets (500 mg each), if aspirin is not tolerated.

Dihydrocodeine (DF 118), 30-60 mg.

Compound codeine tablets (Aspirin, phenacetin and codeine soluble tablets, B.P.) or Codis (codeine and aspirin): Codeine is liable to cause constipation.

Propoxyphene (Distalgesic = propoxyphene and paracetamol; Napsalgesic = propoxyphene and aspirin).

For *moderately severe pain,* something stronger is needed such as Dipipanone (Diconal = dipipanone and cyclizine).

Dextromoramide (Palfium) 5 to 10 mg.

Even stronger are the morphine analogues:

Methadone (Physeptone) 5 to 10 mg.

Levorphanol (Dromoran) 1.5-4.5 mg.

(Pethidine is not recommended).

*More severe pain* needs the *morphine* group, of which the best is diamorphine (heroin).

The side-effects of morphine are important — nausea, sweating, vomiting, drowsiness, respiratory depression and suppression of cough (with consequent liability to chest infection), constipation. Heroin is markedly superior in avoiding vomiting and constipation. Prolonged use of morphine and many of its synthetic analogues (pethidine etc. – see above) ultimately lowers the patient's morale and impairs his mental faculties.

To counter nausea and vomiting, the phenothiazines are useful – perphenazine (Fentazin), prochlorperazine (Stemetil) or chlorpromazine (Largactil). *Chlorpromazine* is particularly useful. Besides potentiating the analgesic effect of other drugs and exerting an anti-emetic influence, it helps to control disturbed and confused patients, including those with raised intracranial pressure from cerebral metastases. It is deservedly popular with ward nurses, and can be given either by mouth (25-50 mg t.d.s.) as tablets or syrup, or by intramuscular injection; large doses, e.g. 300 mg a day can be given if necessary.

One of the most favoured and effective prescriptions is the famous *Brompton Mixture* (devised at the Brompton Hospital, London) – morphine hydrochloride 5-15 mg, cocaine hydrochloride 10 mg, gin 4 ml, honey 4 ml, chloroform water to 15 ml. The dose of morphine can begin at 5 mg and be increased as necessary. Heroin can with advantage be substituted for morphia, working upwards from 2.5 mg. It is certainly the best drug for resistant pain and also for persistent cough. One advantage of giving a mixture by mouth is that the dosage of the constituents can be increased in subsequent bottles without rousing the fears of a suspicious patient who might be worried by an increased number of tablets. There is now an excellent B.P.C. (British Pharmaceutical Codex) formulation – Elixir of diamorphine, cocaine and chlorpromazine; a 5 ml dose contains 5 mg heroin and the heroin dosage can be adjusted down or up as necessary.

Some nurses and doctors are surprisingly reluctant to use morphia and heroin – perhaps out of a vague fear of addiction. But at this stage of disease, this is no problem at all. Certainly they should not be given in unnecessarily large doses or merely to cloud consciousness. Small but frequent dosage should be the golden rule, just enough to break the vicious circle of expectation of pain. It is astonishing how effective this treatment can be and bring a seemingly moribund patient even to positive enjoyment of the last few weeks or months of life.

It may be necessary to try various drugs and doses before the right regime is found. The minimum needed for analgesia should be used, for excessive dosage makes the patient 'dopey' and demoralised. Oral administration may be satisfactory to the end. Parenteral treatment may eventually be indicated – beginning with 10 mg morphine sulphate subcutaneously (or 5 mg diamorphine hydrochloride) and working upwards as necessary. A useful alternative is the long-acting Duromorph, a microcrystalline suspension of morphine injected twice daily. In any event, single doses of morphine should never exceed 60 mg. If more is needed, it is better to give more sedatives and tranquillisers, such as amylobarbitone (Amytal) 30 mg, or phenobarbitone 30-60 mg, or chlorpromazine (above). Suppositories may be just as good as injections, e.g.

oxycodone pectinate (Proladone), one or two every 6-8 hours.

Skin rashes may occur and be relieved by an anti-histamine, e.g. promethazine hydrochloride (Phenergan) 10-50 mg daily in single or divided doses, or chlorpheniramine (Piriton) 4-16 mg daily.

*Hypnotics* are usually indicated: insomnia is demoralising. The choice is again wide, e.g.:

Chloral hydrate 1-1.5 g (chloral mixture B.P.C.).

Dichlorphenazone (Welldorm) 650-1300 mg (or as elixir).

Pentobarbitone 100-200 mg.

Glutethamide (Doriden) 250-500 mg.

Nitrazepam (Mogadon) 5-10 mg.

*Alcohol* is valuable and need not be denied or restricted. A bedside bottle of whisky or brandy can be a great comfort, and assist sedation and sleep.

*Other Drugs* of use include tricyclic *antidepressants* (amitryptiline, Tryptizol) and benzodiazepine *tranquillisers* (diazepam, Valium).

*Surgical relief of pain.* This is worth considering if life expectancy is not too short.

*Visceral pain*

a. Colostomy (for rectal pain).

b. Relief of ureteric obstruction, by transplantation of ureter(s) or even nephrectomy.

c. Drainage of pus, e.g. pyometra.

d. Sympathectomy, lumbar or sacral; or paravertebral sympathetic nerve block, e.g. coeliac plexus or splanchnic block. Phenol or absolute alcohol is injected, the needle entering at the side of the vertebral column, on one or both sides.


*Somatic pain*

a. Peripheral nerve block, using 5-8 per cent phenol or (even more efficient) chloro-cresol. Intercostal, brachial and cervical blocks are possible. The branches of the fifth (trigeminal) nerve can be injected as they emerge from the skull. Gasserian ganglion block is also feasible but leads to a dry eye and anaesthetic cornea, with risk of corneal ulceration.

b. Intrathecal subarachnoid injection of phenol etc. The sensory fibres of the posterior roots or cauda equina are more affected than the motor nerves. This is most useful for pain below the level of the first lumbar root, though in skilled hands it can be valuable at much higher levels, even cervical. Sphincter paralysis, especially of bladder, may occur, but usually soon recovers. Relief may last up to several months, and injections can be repeated.

c. Epidural injection of a long-lasting oily anaesthetic solution, e.g. into the spinal canal through the sacro-coccygeal membrane for prolonged caudal anaesthesia, or in the cervico-dorsal region for pain in the arm and neck from apical lung tumours (Pancoast tumour).

d. Neuro-surgical procedures, of which the most valuable is

(antero-lateral) *cordotomy* for section of the sensory fibres of the spino-thalamic tract, on one or both sides. Pain and temperature sensation is lost, but touch is retained. Temporary disturbances of bladder and rectum, and weakness of legs, may occur, especially after bilateral section.

A recent advance is *percutaneous electric cordotomy;* under local anaesthesia and X-ray control, an electrode is inserted at cervical level into the antero-lateral tract of the cord, and the nerve fibres destroyed by an electric current. This is very useful for a debilitated patient, unfit for general anaesthesia. Cordotomy should be considered in any case where life expectancy is thought to exceed six months.

Section of cranial nerves is possible, but not often advisable. Section of posterior roots in the spinal canal after partial laminectomy can be valuable, especially at intercostal levels.

## Other symptoms

*Vomiting* is very common and may be intractable. There may be a psychological element, owing to pain and apprehension; if these are relieved, vomiting may cease or at least be controllable by anti-emetics (see above). The diet may be at fault, and antacids may help. Soda-water and iced water are usually tolerated when nothing else is.

If mechanical obstruction is responsible, an intragastric tube and suction may be required. Fluid intake must be maintained to prevent dehydration. Intravenous drip should rarely be necessary and rectal tap-water is simpler and generally adequate.

*Dysphagia* is always distressing, and the patient may be terrified of choking to death. Mechanical obstruction (e.g. in oesophageal or lung cancer) or extreme soreness may demand an intragastric tube (via the nose) or even justify the surgical insertion of a Mousseau-Barbin or Celestin tube (see p. 146).

In mouth or throat cancer, soreness may be helped by aspirin mucilage, benzocaine lozenges, Mucaine or Xylocaine Viscous Solution. Frequent mouth washes and local anaesthetic sprays are useful.

Fluid is more important than food, and nutrition can be maintained for months by liquid Complan and vitamin supplements, etc.

Gastrostomy or jejunostomy should very rarely be considered – it is usually a very doubtful blessing.

In terminal patients, dry mouths are common, liable to monilial infection (thrush), which should be confirmed by a swab. Treatment is by nystatin as a local paint and/or tablets to deal with infection elsewhere in the alimentary tract. Gentian violet ($\frac{1}{2}$ per cent aqueous solution) is also useful locally. A sore red tongue may respond to nicotinamide tablets (50 mg).

*Dyspnoea,* if due to bronchial spasm, needs relaxant drugs (ephedrine, aminophylline, atropine). It is a common problem in lung cancer, and a bedside oxygen cylinder with a face mask may give relief (even if only psychological). Putting the bed near an open window may be equally effective.

Persistent cough needs diamorphine linctus, and infected sputum may be controlled by antibiotics.

Respiratory obstruction, from growths of larynx, pharynx etc. justifies tracheostomy to relieve the intolerable fear of suffocation.

*Constipation* is of continual interest and worry both to patients and relatives. They should be assured that a daily bowel movement is neither essential nor important. Purgatives should be banned, but gentle laxatives (liquid paraffin emulsion, Senokot tablets or granules) or suppositories are useful, to avoid the need for enemas which are exhausting for the patient. If faecal inpaction threatens, enemas may be needed.

*Urinary incontinence* may call for an indwelling catheter plus a urinary antiseptic drug, e.g. nitrofurantoin (Furadantin).

Urinary fistula (e.g. vesico-vaginal) may justify diversion — transplantation of ureters into the colon (the risk of ascending pyelonephritis and electrolyte disturbances can be ignored in the circumstances) or an ileal conduit (see p. 155).

*Faecal incontinence* is less troublesome than urinary incontinence provided there is no diarrhoea. Colostomy is often indicated especially if there is rectal pain (but radiation enteritis may make colostomy a curse).

*Bed-sores* — like so many other things — are better prevented than treated. The most important prophylactics are dryness of the skin and frequent changes of position. Patients should be encouraged to be mobile as long as possible, and to be out of bed part of the time. Pressure points, especially sacrum and heels, should be protected by two-hourly changes of position. If dry, they should be rubbed with alcohol; if infected, eusol. dressings are applied. It is particularly important to control incontinence if at all possible. Rubber rings, sheepskin rugs and ripple beds are all valuable.

## Terminal care

The care of the dying is, of course, not confined to cancer, but cancer does provide the bulk of the trying problems involved.

The subject of death hardly appears in any but the most perfunctory manner in training curricula. Perhaps this is not surprising, with our emphasis on curative (and now preventive) medicine, but it has as much claim to be regarded as a specialty as many others. 'Thanatology' (Greek thanatos = death) sounds repulsive, but a process that affects everyone cannot be unworthy of serious attention. It would not be going too far to insist that the dignity and comfort of the dying are better criteria of the quality of a civilisation than the sophistication of the computerised electronic gadgetry of the most expensive intensive-care unit.

*Place of death.* This will naturally vary with the available resources, social and economic pattern etc., especially the cohesion of family life. In the extended family, with the generations and near relatives living together, the problems and solutions will differ from those of the small family unit where a high value is put on privacy, and where employment of most or all adults outside the home is common. In western countries, especially U.S.A., social mobility and rootlessness are increasing; and the picture differs between urban and rural communities, large and small towns, cosmopolitan ports and mining villages, etc.

Any figures about cancer patients as a whole can only be rough generalisations, but in England the following apply at the present time:

a. Five to ten per cent never reach hospital at all. This is especially true of the old and frail (over 70) and particularly for gastric cancer. Some refuse treatment, others are simply too senile.

b. Five per cent die of causes other than their cancers, especially cardiovascular.

c. Twenty-five per cent need only simple medical care. They are fortunate in fading away fairly peacefully, with increasing weakness but no serious pain.

d. Fifty per cent die at home. The family doctor and visiting nurse cope with terminal care, backed by the relatives.

e. Ten to fifteen per cent need hospital care in the terminal stages.

The point where curative efforts and the intention to prolong life cease, and terminal care can be said to begin, is usually clear enough. The boundary, however, is becoming more blurred and difficult to decide with the advent of new techniques such as cytotoxic drugs, heroic surgery (e.g. pelvic exenteration), transplants, etc. There is a famous couplet:

> Thou shalt not kill, but need'st not strive
> Officiously to keep alive.

It was meant ironically, but does point to what is often felt to be a dilemma. For example, in hopless cases it is unwise to transfuse for severe anaemia or haemorrhage, or prescribe antibiotics for bronchopneumonia or anticoagulants for thrombosis. The overriding considerations must always be — the interest and comfort of the patient. This is easy to say, but does not mean that the patient's best interest is always obvious or will appear identical to two equally competent and honest practitioners. But in practice, the more experienced the doctor, the less difficulty does he find in deciding when to call a halt (and to restrain the well-meant enthusiasm of his junior assistants). As Lord Horder put it — 'The good doctor is aware of the distinction between prolonging life and prolonging the act of dying.' And he will not succumb to the blandishments of mere technique in the face of charity.*

*Euthanasia* or 'mercy killing' is apt to be discussed in this context. A bill was recently brought before Parliament to legalise this, but was rejected. It is a logically attractive and well-intentioned idea, but the

---

* One observer is alleged to have said 'No one nowadays is allowed to die without being cured'.

dangers and drawbacks are at least as obvious as the advantages. *Not many doctors would be willing to partake in any such official scheme. No doctor worthy of the name prolongs misery unnecessarily, and any widespread demand for legalised euthanasia would reflect a lack of confidence and trust in the available medical services. The word means 'a quiet and easy death', and if we do not take steps to ensure this, then we have failed in one (and not the least) of the supreme duties of care owed to our patients.

The burden of terminal care is not always willingly shouldered, especially by those whose training is so markedly orientated to curative medicine. It may even be felt as a reproach, as a burden of guilt. This is surely wrong, even immoral and selfish. The wards of a general acute hospital, it is true, are not the right places for such care. They are too busy, the hectic tempo and environment are quite unsuitable, and death has a bad effect on the morale of other patients. Radiotherapy wards are liable to have a relatively high proportion of patients with a very poor prognosis. If the terminal stage must be on the ward, the patient should be in a side-ward if possible.

This is a time for particular consideration not only for the patient but for his relatives, who often need as much sympathy and support as the patient. One thing needful is so often difficult to give, but of the highest importance – time; time for the patient to unburden himself, to reveal his many worries and fears. Too often he will suffer in silence, afraid to impose on busy nurses and doctors, afraid of pain and loneliness and the unknown. It is not so much death itself he fears, but the process of dying. If only he can have the opportunity of a ready and willing ear, this alone will go a long way to ease his burden. In fact, one of the most important services which nurses and doctors can provide is to give the patient the chance to unload his worries on to them. He should be given every opportunity to talk, and never to think we have insufficient time for him. If only he will voice his fears, something can almost always be done to alleviate if not remove them. In this respect, nurses are often in a better position than the doctor to discover the cause of a patient's anxiety, and either deal with it herself or call in the appropriate person to do so.

The services of relatives, clergymen, social workers, solicitors (to make a will) etc. should be made available as required.

The religious element will be of prime importance to some, and of little or none to others. But whatever our own personal views may be about possible life after death, our words and actions should at the very least not appear to contradict this possibility and hope.

Many, even most, patients die at home – and home is the place preferred by most patients and is the ideal place if circumstances (and

---

*The tale is told of two doctors who in their youth made a pact, that the first to be in serious trouble would be put out of his misery by the other. The years passed, with their accompaniment of human troubles. Came the day when both doctors gave instructions that the other was not in future to be admitted to his house under any circumstances.

relatives) are suitable. But the stress on the family is sometimes more than they should be called on to bear. Hospital accommodation is usually very difficult to find at this stage. Much can be done by district nurses, home helps, night sitters and the family doctor, yet there is a great need for special units devoted to terminal care. A few such already exist. Some of the best of them are owed – not surprisingly – to religious inspiration, and the churches have set an historic example in this field, which should be more widely followed by the State. Not every nurse or doctor will feel called to this type of work, but it has its own rewards and satisfactions, and the word 'euthanasia' ought properly to become associated with this – i.e. mercy-dying – rather than its conventional sense of mercy-killing.

Some practical points for the final stage, culled from experienced nurses, may be useful:

a. The patient should be allowed to find his own most comfortable position. Most prefer to be propped up and to see around them.

b. Vision weakens. Good lighting and open curtains should be the rule.

c. Thirst is often prominent, even in the absence of pain. The mouth and lips should be kept moist, even in apparent unconsciousness.

d. Hearing is often acute. Conversation in his presence should be guarded, and a relative or priest should, if appropirate, be present at the end.

e. The distressing death rattle may be relieved by an injection of atropine.

f. If at home, the family should be prepared for likely crises, e.g. vomiting or haemorrhage – which can be alarming and even terrifying. They should be told what to expect, and what actions need to be taken concerning death certification, cremation, undertakers, etc.

# Envoi: Optimism and Pessimism in Cancer

*We dance around in a ring and suppose,*
*But the Secret sits in the middle and knows.*

Robert Frost

The preceding chapters have tried to hold the balance between unhelpful pessimism and unjustified optimism. The image of cancer in the lay mind, especially at the lower end of the social scale, tends to be one of complete incurability and practically certain death. And it is widely believed that cancer is the commonest cause of death. (Actually it is the second commonest cause, and cardiovascular deaths are almost twice as common.) This is bad enough, even if understandable. What is equally disturbing, however, is the image in the minds of some nurses and doctors. Recent surveys among medical students, general practitioners and nurses revealed a significant degree of pessimism regarding the prognosis even of early cancer in various sites (e.g. cervix, seminoma of testis) where the prognosis is in fact distinctly favourable, with lasting cures of 70 per cent or more. Pessimism was most pronounced among the nurses. This is particularly significant, in view of their influence as agents of public education. Between a pessimistic doctor and a pessimistic nurse, the apprehensive patient is in an unenviable position indeed.

Both pessimism and optimism can be justified — it depends on the point of view. True, the majority of cancers are still fatal. But in this country about 30 000 cancer cures are now achieved every year. And the lethality of cancer (i.e. the death-rate in particular age groups) in most sites is gradually declining, with the striking exception of lung cancer.

It is, of course, not mysterious that nurses should be inclined to pessimism. So much of the losing battles falls to them to fight. Successful cases need little or no further nursing care, but the failures often remain taxing problems to the end. What is less justifiable is the attitude of some doctors, especially in hospitals. Medicine to them means 'curative' medicine, and if cure is impossible they feel somehow affronted and embarrassed, stricken as if by a guilt complex, and hasten to relieve themselves of the burden of further care. Nothing is more demoralising to a patient than to think that the doctor responsible for his previous treatment has washed his hands of him.

All those, nurses or doctors, who undertake the care of the cancer patient, need to add a pinch of optimism to enhance the flavour of their work, and to give moral as well as physical support to the patient. If they cannot, their talents are better employed elsewhere.

In the modern era, cancer therapy began with surgery. Radiation came later, and the two have remained the mainstays of treatment. Both agents have now probably approached or reached their technical limits, with the possible exception of transplant surgery. Chemotherapy has made a limited but significant contribution, and still has some way to go – no one can say how far, though if it can join hands with molecular biology its contribution could yet be dazzling. Emerging from the shade now comes the promise of immunotherapy; expectations are keen, but much fundamental work has still to be done. Beyond this it is fruitless to peer.

A recent forecast of possible future trends in medicine was made by an expert group of doctors, research workers, pharmacologists and others. Their conclusions about cancer were as follows:*

Problems in this field are rated at best as difficult and at worst as extremely difficult. There is unanimity in the forecasts that the basic difficulties reside in the multiplicity of causes and types of cancer, in the fact that there are probably many points in the relevant cell processes where dysfunction can occur, and in the very complex nature of those processes.

The fact that experiments cannot be carried out in man provides another difficulty, especially in relation to cancers caused by viruses. Another major difficulty in the way of advances in the field of cytotoxic cancer therapy is that of finding an agent that will both harm cancer cells and leave adjacent healthy cells untouched.

One forecast suggests that accidental observations in fields other than that of cancer are more likely to yield fruitful therapeutic results than planned cancer research; and various of the less optimistic forecasts suggest that earlier diagnosis of cancer, and skilful and highly selective combinations of surgery, radiotherapy, immunochemistry and chemotherapy will provide such improvements as are to be attained in this field by 1990. Total organ transplants are seen as one feasible answer to certain cancers: medicines will then be reserved to deal with any secondary cancers while they are still small. According to this group of conservative forecasts, there is likely to be a number of anti-cancer compounds developed, not just one 'wonder' cancer cure.

A gloomy view expressed by some is that new cancers will emerge, possibly as fast as existing ones are dealt with, and that these new cancers will prove extremely difficult to control.

However, the more optimistic forecasts predict that by the 1980s we shall have achieved, via studies of cell metabolism and genetics, an understanding of the basic processes controlling cell division, and of how chemical, viral, and hormonal carcinogens fit into this process; and we shall have discovered various new factors that can alter the process,

* I am indebted to the Office of Health Economics, London, for permission to include this extract from their booklet, *Medicines in the 1990's: A Technological Forecast* (1969).

more particularly those that are now presumed to be responsible for cancers whose causation is obscure. Following these advances in knowledge, campaigns of prevention will be possible and ways should have been found to make such campaigns more effective than the present one against cigarette smoking. There will also be a variety of therapies for established cancer. It is suggested that by 1990, 70 per cent of cancers will be controllable.

Perhaps we should echo the sentiment of that early Father of the Church, Tertullian:

*It is certain because it is impossible*

From the same group of forecasts comes the suggestion that work on the immune aspects of graft rejection, and on immune responses to certain cancers may also produce quite rapid results. Indeed, both specific and non-specific means of stimulating the body's immune responses (i.e. in this context its cancer-rejection mechanism) are foreseen by 1980.

By 1980, the same more optimistic prophets say, we shall have made some progress with possibly naturally occurring anti-cancer compounds which will be specific to particular types of tumour. It may well happen that the discovery of such new compounds will, if they are specific enough, indicate the aetiology of a particular cancer, which will lead to the development of more accurate research models and so in time to the development of further new anti-cancer medicines, even more powerful or specific. Again, while only a few cancers will be shown to be caused by viruses, means of stimulating immunity to the antigens of the responsible viruses are foreseen as being available by 1990. And lasty from the hopeful group comes the suggestion that fruitful work on enzymes, will be carried out between 1970 and 1990.

# Appendix

# Some Word Derivations

*The meaning of anything is usually another word for the same thing.*

Sir Charles Chaplin

Medical vocabulary contains a vast quantity of complex words, much of it jargon (politely called 'technical terminology'). It derives mostly from Greek and Latin, and naturally embodies a good deal of medical and other history – a fascinating hobby in itself. On a more unilitarian level, it is both illuminating and helpful to understand the root meanings especially of the more complicated constructions, which otherwise are apt to sound mere gibberish.

For instance, how does one react to dysdiadochokinesis, bothryomyces, phlyctenular? It is at least interesting to know that malaria simply means 'bad air' (supposed to cause the disease) and quarantine means 'forty (days)'. Even the average classical scholar would be hard put to gather the meaning of many medical words without a little research. Hardly any nurses and very few doctors will be classical scholars today.

Some derivations have been given in the text. Here we add a few more that need a rather longer explanation, mostly concerning the intracranial tumours mentioned in Chapter 9. With a few exceptions, they are all from the Greek.

*Oma* is a word-ending denoting a tumour or abnormal growth. Compare 'osis' meaning a state or condition, and 'itis' which originally referred to any disease process but is now restricted to inflammation.
*Pituitary.* Pituita (Latin) = mucus or phlegm. Nasal secretion was thought to come through the skull from the base of the brain.

The gland is a composite structure and its cells react differently to histological stains.
*Chromophobe* cells are averse to stains. Chroma = colour; phobos = fear.
*Eosinophil* cells take up acid stains, hence their alternative name 'acidophil'. Philos means loving; eosin is a rose-coloured dye (eos = dawn).
*Basophil* cells take up basic stains; acids and bases are chemical opposites.
*Acromegaly* is the disease syndrome associated with excessive hormonal secretion from eosinophil cells. Patients develop enlarged hands, feet, jaw

etc. Acron = tip, extremity; mega = large (compare megavoltage, hepatomegaly etc.).

*Glioma.* Glia = glue. Neuroglia ('nerve glue') is the specialised connective tissue or binding cells of the central nervous system.

*Astrocytoma.* Astron = star, cytos = receptacle, cell. The microscopic appearance of the cell is star-shaped.

*Ependymoma.* Ependyma = garment. The name was given by the great 19th century German pathologist Virchow to the lining membrane of the cerebral ventricles and central canal of the spinal cord.

*Medulloblastoma.* Latin medulla = marrow, from 'medius' = middle. It denotes the inner part or marrow of an organ, but in this case refers to a particular part of the back of the brain (the cerebellar region). It corresponds to Greek 'myelos', as in myeloma, myeloid leukaemia etc. Blastos = sprout, shoot, germ – i.e. the parent of the mature cell.

*Oligodendroglioma.* Oligos = few or small; dendron = tree. Oligodendroglia refers to cells of the neuroglia which have relatively few and short branches.

*Pinealoma.* Latin pinus = pine-cone. The pineal body is a cone-shaped structure behind the third ventricle.

*Paraplegia.* Para = by the side of; the primary meaning refers to position, as in parathyroid (alongside the thyroid) or parametrium (alongside the uterus: Greek metra = womb). Plegia = blow or stroke. The name was originally applied to a stroke involving one side, now called hemiplegia (hemi = half), but was later used to refer to involvement of the lower limbs.

A secondary meaning of para is: to one side, amiss, faulty or irregular – as in paraesthesia, i.e. disturbance of feeling.

*Teratoma.* Tera = monster or misshapen organism.

# Further Reading

*Another damned, thick, square book! Always
scribble, scribble, eh! Mr. Gibbon.*
                              Duke of Gloucester (1743-1805)

**General and Historical**
Curie, E. *Madame Curie.* Various editions, e.g. (1962) London: Heinemann. (1959) New
    York: Pocket Books. (Biography of the discoverer of radium, by her daughter.)
Reid, R. (1974) *Marie Curie* London: Collins.
Donizetti, P. (1967) *Shadow and Substance, The Story of Medical Radiography.* Oxford:
    Pergamon Press (also includes radiotherapy).
Roberts, ff. (1966). *Medical Terms: Their Origin and Construction* 4th edn. London:
    Heinemann.

**Cancer**
For the 'intelligent layman':
Harris, R. J. C. (1975) *Cancer,* revised edition. Penguin Books.
Harris, R. J. C. (ed.) (1970 *What We Know about Cancer.* London: Allen & Unwin.
Brooke, B. N. (1971) *Understanding Cancer.* London: Heinemann.
Wilkinson, J. (1973) *The Conquest of Cancer.* London: Hart-Davis, Macgibbon.

*For doctors*
Ackerman, L. V. & Del Regato, J. A. (1970) *Cancer: Diagnosis, Treatment, Prognosis,*
    4th edn. St. Louis, Mo.: Mosby Co.; London: Kimpton.
Moore, C. (1970) *Synopsis of Clinical Cancer,* 2nd edn. St. Louis, Mo.: Mosby Co.; Lon-
    don: Kimpton.
Nealon, T. F. (ed.) (1965) *Management of the Patient With Cancer.* Philadelphia and
    London: Saunders.
*Cancer Management* (A Special Graduate Course sponsored by the American Cancer
    Society) (1968) Philadelphia: Lippincott; London: Pitman Medical.
Raven, R. W. & Roe, F. J. C. (ed.) (1967) *The Prevention of Cancer* London:
    Butterworths.
Ashley (D. J. B.) (1972) *An Introduction to the General Pathology of Tumours* Bristol:
    Wright. (Short-Recommended to nurses also).

**Cancer nursing**
Publications of the American Cancer Society, New York:
    *Essentials of Cancer Nursing.*
    *A Cancer Source Book for Nurses.*
Capra, C. G. (1972) *The Care of the Cancer Patient* London: Heinemann.
Deeley, T. J. (1970) *A Guide to Radiotherapy Nursing* Edinburgh: Livingstone.
Saunders, C. (1967), *The Management of Terminal Illness* London: Hospital Medicine
    Publications. (A short pamphlet. Recommended. The author is qualified both as nurse
    and doctor.)
Raven, R. W. (ed.) (1970) *Domiciliary Care of the Patient with Cancer.* London:
    Heinemann.

Raven, R. W. (ed.) (1972) *Rehabilitation of the Cancer Disabled.* London: Heinemann.
Deeley, T. J. et al. (1974) *Guide to Oneological Nursing* Edinburgh: Churchill Livingstone.

## Radiotherapy

Walter, J., Miller, H. Bomford, K. & Neal, F.E. (in press), *Short Textbook of Radiotherapy 4th edn.* Edinburgh: Churchill Livingstone.
Barnes, P. A. & Rees, D. J. (1972). *A Concise Textbook of Radiotherapy* London: Faber and Faber. (Similar in scope.)
Lowry, S. (1974) *Fundamentals of Radiation Therapy* London: English Universities Press.
Rafla, S & Rotman, M. (1974) *Introduction to Radiotherapy* St Louis: C. V. Mosby Co.

*For medical radiotherapists*
Moss, W. T., Brand, W. N & Battifora, H. (1973) *Radiation Oncology.* 4th edn. St Louis: C. V. Mosby Co.
Fletcher, G. H. (ed) (1973) *Textbook of Radiotheapy* 2nd edn. Philadelphia: Lea and Febiger; London: Kimpton.
Paterson, R. (1963) *Treatment of Malignant Disease by Radiotherapy* 2nd edn. London: Arnold.

## Isotopes

For the 'intelligent layman':
Putnam, J. L. (1965) *Isotopes* 2nd edn. Penguin Books.

*Medical*
*Diagnostic Use of Radioisotopes in Medicine* (1969) London: Hospital Medicine Publications. (A short pamphlet.)
Maynard, C. D. (ed.) (1969) *Clinical Nuclear Medicine* Philadelphia: Lea and Febiger.
Barnaby, C. F. (1969) *Radionuclides in Medicine* London: Souvenir Press.
Wagner, H. N. & Block, I. (ed.) (1975) *Nuclear Medicine* New York: Hospital Practice.
Oliver, R. (1971) *Principles of the Use of Radio-isotope Tracers in Clinical and Research Investigation.* Oxford: Pergamon Press.

## Radiation Biology and Hazards

Alexander, P. (1965) *Atomic Radiation and Life* 2nd edn. Penguin Books. (Recommended.)
Coggle, J. E. (1971) *Biological Effects of Radiation.* London & Winchester: Wykeham Publications.
Mayneord, W. V. (1964) *Radiation and Health* Nuffield Provincial Hospitals Trust. (Well written short survey of the chief problems.)
Hersey, J. *Hiroshima* various editions, e.g. (1966) New York: Bantam Books. School edition, London: Hamilton. (Graphic account of the effects of the atom bomb.)
*The Safe Use of Ionising Radiations. A Handbook for Nurses* H.M.S.O. (Should be read by all nurses concerned with radiation work.)

## Cytotoxic drugs

Short accounts will be found in books on Drugs and Pharmacology for Nurses etc. The following are for doctors:
Greenwald, E. S. (1973) *Cancer Chemotherapy* 2nd edn. London: Kimpton.
Boesen, E. & Davis, W. (1969). *Cytotoxic Drugs in the Treatment of Cancer,* London: Arnold.
Cole, W. H. (1970) *Chemotheapy of Cancer* London: Kimpton.
Holland, J. F. & Frei, E. (ed.) (1973) *Cancer Medicine* Philadelphia: Lea & Febiger.
Cline, M. J. & Haskell, C. M. (1975) *Cancer Chemotherapy.* 2nd edn. Philadelphia: Saunders.

# Index

PRINTED BY HUNTSMEN OFFSET PRINTING (PTE) LTD.